ESSENTIALS OF VETERINARY ANATOMY AND PHYSIOLOGY

For Elsevier:

Senior Commissioning Editor: Mary Seager
Development Editors: Catharine Steers/
                                    Rita Demetriou-Swanwick
Project Manager: Jane Dingwall, Andrew Palfreyman
Design: Andrew Chapman / Stewart Larking

ESSENTIALS OF VETERINARY ANATOMY AND PHYSIOLOGY

Victoria Aspinall, BVSc MRCVS
Director, Abbeydale Vetlink Veterinary
Training Ltd, Gloucester, UK

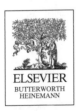

ELSEVIER
BUTTERWORTH
HEINEMANN

Edinburgh London New York Oxford Philadelphia St Louis
Sydney Toronto 2005

ELSEVIER
BUTTERWORTH
HEINEMANN

First published 2005

ISBN 0 7506 8802 5

British Library Cataloguing in Publication Data
A catalogue record for this book is available from the British Library

Library of Congress Cataloging in Publication Data
A catalog record for this book is available from the Library of Congress

your source for books, journals and multimedia in the health sciences

www.elsevierhealth.com

The publisher's policy is to use paper manufactured from sustainable forests

Printed in China

Contents

Preface

Essentials of Veterinary Anatomy and Physiology has been written to provide a form of quick reference to underpin more detailed texts on the subject of anatomy and physiology. Each chapter covers one body system and clearly outlines such important points as its functions and parts and then goes on to describe the main anatomical features and the physiology of those parts. Extensive use is made of bullet points, lists and tables so that the facts are easily accessible. The number of diagrams is limited to those that are entirely necessary to explain a particularly complicated structure but it is felt that this adds to the simplified format rather than detracting from it. Everyone has 'memory black spots' or facts they find difficult to learn and remember and it is hoped that the 'Memory Joggers' distributed throughout the text will introduce the student to ways in which to memorise them. However, it should be pointed out that everyone learns in a different way so these 'Memory Joggers' are only suggestions and it may be better for the student to invent their own mnemonics, lists or catchy phrases. As the anatomy and physiology of each system is inextricably linked with that of other systems, references to other relevant chapters in the book have been included so that the student can quickly turn to the correct area without having to consult the Index or Contents page. As seen previously in *Introduction to Veterinary Anatomy and Physiology* (Aspinall and O'Reilly), exotic species have also been included and these chapters have been used to compare their varying anatomy with that of the dog and cat.

Essentials of Veterinary Anatomy and Physiology is designed to be of use primarily to veterinary nursing students and to this end it closely follows the syllabus for the veterinary nursing course; however, it will also be invaluable to students of animal care and animal science at all levels and even to first year veterinary students who need to remind themselves of the underpinning facts.

There are many texts on the anatomy and physiology of the dog and the cat but for some time there has been a need for a book supplying quick reminders of the facts, and I hope that this is what *Essentials of Veterinary Anatomy and Physiology* will provide.

Victoria Aspinall 2004.

Acknowledgements

This book is dedicated to my patient husband Richard and to my children, Charlie, William, Nico and Polly, and also to my numerous cats and dogs who not only let me use them as anatomical specimens but also keep me fit by always wanting to be let out (or in) the moment that I sit down at my computer! Writing a book is an all-consuming occupation and they have all learnt to thrive on neglect.

I would also like to thank all those at Elsevier in particular Mary Seager for her unfailing support and backup, and Catharine Steers and Rita Demetriou-Swanwick.

1
First Principles

Anatomy – the study of the structure of the body and its tissues.
Physiology – the study of the function of the body and its tissues.
Histology – the microscopic study of the body tissues.
Pathology – the study of the effect disease has on the body tissues.
Histopathology – the microscopic study of the effect disease has on the body tissues.

CLASSIFICATION

All living creatures are classified or arranged into groups of similar species related by their common evolutionary ancestry, so that their complex forms and their inter-relationships can be understood. Imagine sorting a pack of cards into piles related by the type of suit or by numbers – this is what happens when animals are classified. The study of classification is known as **taxonomy**.

All organisms are divided into five **kingdoms**. These are:
- Animalia – multicellular animals
- Plantae – plants
- Monera – prokaryotic unicellular organisms, e.g. bacteria and blue-green algae
- Protista – eukaryotic unicellular and simple multicellular organisms, e.g. protozoa
- Fungi – eukaryotic organisms that reproduce by forming spores.

In veterinary practice we are principally interested in the members of the Animal Kingdom but we must not forget that many disease-causing organisms or pathogens come from other kingdoms.

Each kingdom is divided into smaller and smaller groups, each of which contains progressively fewer organisms. Thus, the first group, the **phylum**, contains a wide variety of organisms that have a few basic features in common but have a great many differences. However, the organisms in a **genus** are very similar and those of the same **species** are identical in appearance. In descending order, the groups are known as:

- **phylum** (plural phyla)
- **class**
- **order**
- **family**
- **genus** (plural genera)
- **species**

For greater scientific clarification, these groups may be subdivided. For example, a phylum may be broken up into several subphyla. The mammals of veterinary importance are all within the following groups:

Phylum: Chordata – all have a backbone
Class: Mammalia – covered in fur and suckle their young with milk
Order:
1. Carnivora – flesh-eaters, e.g. dogs and cats
2. Rodentia – have incisors with persistent pulp cavities, e.g. mice and gerbils
3. Lagomorpha – have two pairs of upper incisors, e.g. rabbits
4. Perissodactyla – are hoofed and bear weight on an odd number of toes, e.g. horses
5. Artiodactyla – are hoofed and bear weight on an even number of toes, e.g. cattle, sheep and deer.

Table 1.1 shows examples of how some companion animals are classified.

Animals are normally referred to by their genus and species, e.g. *Canis familiaris*, the domestic dog. This system of having two names, known as the **binomial system**, was invented by the Swedish botanist Carl von Linné or Linnaeus (1707–1778). The genus and species should be written in italics with a capital initial letter for the genus and a small initial letter for the species, e.g. *Felis catus*, the domestic cat. The generic name is

| Table 1.1 | Classification of some common species of companion animals | | | | |

	Dog	**Cat**	**Rabbit**	**Garter Snake**	**Budgerigar**
Kingdom	Animalia	Animalia	Animalia	Animalia	Animalia
Phylum	Chordata	Chordata	Chordata	Chordata	Chordata
Class	Mammalia	Mammalia	Mammalia	Reptilia	Aves
Order	Carnivora	Carnivora	Lagomorpha	Squamata	Psittaciformes
Sub-order	-	-	-	Serpentes	-
Family	Canidae	Felidae	Leporidae	Colubridae	Psittacidae
Genus	*Canis*	*Felis*	*Oryctolagus*	*Thamnophis*	*Melopsittacus*
Species	*familiaris*	*catus*	*cuniculus*	*sirtalis*	*undulatus*

often modified to form an adjective to describe the characteristics of the animal in question; thus, cats are described as 'feline' and dogs as 'canine'.

A species may be divided into **breeds**, which may be considered to be small samples of a species. Breeds are exhibited by dogs, cats and rabbits. Members of a breed are linked by certain characteristics but they are the same species as members of other breeds. For example, all domestic dogs are *Canis familiaris* but may be divided into such breeds as the Springer Spaniel, Labrador and Yorkshire Terrier. These breeds may be isolated by geography or pedigree, but if they are crossed or interbred they will still produce a healthy fertile representative of *Canis familiaris*, although it may be described as a crossbreed or mongrel.

Memory Jogger

All living organisms can be classified into **k**ingdom, **p**hylum, **c**lass, **o**rder, **f**amily, **g**enus, **s**pecies and sometimes **b**reed. To help you remember this, use the mnemonic 'Keith prefers class over form. Good show, Bertie!'

ANATOMICAL DIRECTIONS

When you are describing the anatomical structure of an animal, it is important to be able to relate the position of one part of an organ or a tissue to that of another. This gives rise to some important terminology:

- DORSAL – towards the back or upper surface of the body, head, neck and tail
- VENTRAL – towards the lower surface or belly of the body, head, neck and tail
- PROXIMAL – the part of a structure that lies closest to the body
- DISTAL – the part of a structure that lies furthest away from the body
- MEDIAL – towards the centre or midline of the body
- LATERAL – towards the side of the body, away from the midline
- SUPERFICIAL – near the surface of the body
- DEEP – closer to the centre of the body
- EXTERNAL – on the outside or closer to the surface than another structure
- INTERNAL – on the inside or closer to the inner depths than another structure
- CRANIAL OR ANTERIOR – closer to the head
- CAUDAL OR POSTERIOR – closer to the tail
- ROSTRAL – towards the nose; used to describe structures on the head
- PALMAR – the undersurface of the forepaw and lower fore-leg; the surface opposite to the upper side, which is the dorsal surface
- PLANTAR – the undersurface of the hind paw and lower hind leg; the surface opposite to the upper side, which is the dorsal surface.

The planes of the body, which divide it into sections, are:
- MEDIAN PLANE – divides the body longitudinally into two equal halves
- SAGITTAL PLANE – any plane that lies parallel to the median plane
- TRANSVERSE PLANE – runs across the body or a limb at right angles to the median plane or long axis.

THE MAMMALIAN CELL

The cell is the basic unit of all living organisms. A cell is able to survive as a free-living entity or, as seen in structures such as in plants and in our familiar animals, groups of cells combine to form the complex tissues and organs that make up the whole body.

- **A tissue** is a collection of cells and their products in which one type of cell predominates, e.g. muscle tissue, nervous tissue.
- **An organ** is a collection of different tissues that work together to perform a particular function. For example, the heart is made of muscle, connective, nervous and epithelial tissues.
- **A system** is a collection of parts, structures, organs and tissues that are linked by their contribution to a common function, e.g. the respiratory system.

CELL STRUCTURE

Although all cells have the same basic structure they can be subdivided into two main types:

- **somatic cells** – most of the cells of the body
- **germ cells or sex cells** – cells involved in the reproductive process, i.e. the ova in the ovaries and the spermatozoa in the testes.

Each cell is a miniature factory that carries out a number of functions fundamental to the survival and effectiveness of the cell. These functions, which include respiration, excretion, nutrition and reproduction, are performed by the different structures that make up the cell.

When a mammalian cell is viewed under a **light microscope** (this is the type of microscope routinely used in veterinary practices, which magnifies up to 1500 times life size), it is possible to see the following structures:

- **Cell or plasma membrane** – a double layer of phospholipid material in which protein molecules are embedded. It acts as a selectively permeable barrier between the internal composition and the external environment, allowing some substances to pass through while others are held back.
- **Cytoplasm** – appears as an amorphous fluid filling the cell. It contains all the **organelles** and dissolved chemicals necessary for cellular function.
- **Nucleus** – a dense mass of deoxyribonucleic acid (DNA) arranged in **chromosomes**, which are the inheritable

material of the cell. It is surrounded by a **nuclear membrane** and is the control centre of the cell. If the nucleus is removed, the cell will die.

When the cell (Fig. 1.1) is examined under an **electron microscope**, which magnifies up to 250, 000 times life size, the cytoplasm can be seen to be filled with many different types of organelle. These are:

- **Mitochondria** – cigar-shaped structures with a folded lining membrane. These are responsible for **cellular respiration**, in which **energy** is extracted from food substances and stored as adenosine triphosphate (ATP) for later use by the cell. Abundant in cells that require large quantities of energy, e.g. skeletal muscle fibres.
- **Ribosomes** – floating free in the cytoplasm. Responsible for **protein synthesis**.
- **Endoplasmic reticulum** – a series of flattened interconnecting cavities and channels lined with membrane.
  - **Rough endoplasmic reticulum** – the walls are lined with ribosomes, giving a rough appearance. Its function is to **transport proteins** synthesised by the ribosomes around the inside of the cell.
  - **Smooth endoplasmic reticulum** – the walls have no ribosomes. Its function is to **synthesise and transport lipids and steroids.**
- **Golgi body** – a stack of flattened sacs in the cytoplasm. Its function is to **modify** some of the **proteins** produced in the cell. Plays a part in the **formation of lysosomes.**
- **Lysosomes** –membranous sacs containing **lysozymes**, which are enzymes that **digest** by phagocytosis material taken into the cell by endocytosis. They may also destroy worn-out organelles and dead cells.
- **Centrosome** – contains a pair of **centrioles**, which are involved in **cellular reproduction**.
- **Cytoplasmic inclusions or inclusion bodies** – these structures may not always be present in a cell. Some are normal, e.g. melanin, a protective pigment, and haemosiderin, which consists of golden granules resulting from the breakdown of haemoglobin in red blood cells. Other inclusions are abnormal and may indicate some form of disease, such as a virus infection.

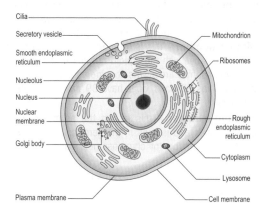

Figure 1.1 A typical animal cell

Memory Jogger
When you are trying to memorise the functions of the parts of the cell, keep it simple and learn it by word association:
* cell membrane – controls what enters and leaves the cell
* nucleus – the control centre or 'brain' of the cell
* mitochondria – energy and cell respiration
* ribosomes – protein synthesis
* endoplasmic reticulum – protein storage and transport.

Exocytosis is the process by which materials are excreted from the cell.
Endocytosis is the process by which materials are taken into the cell. This may be described as:
* **phagocytosis** or cell eating – solid material
* **pinocytosis** or cell drinking – liquids.

CELL GROWTH AND DIVISION

When a body grows or a tissue repairs itself, this is done by increasing the number of cells. A cell grows and when it reaches full size it divides into two, so that one cell becomes two, two cells become four, and so on. The most important part of the cell is the **nucleus**, which is tightly packed with DNA.

The DNA is arranged in pairs of strands, each of which is called a **chromosome**. A resting cell contains the 'diploid' number of chromosomes. These are difficult to differentiate but as the cell prepares to divide they become thicker, denser and more visible.

- **Diploid number** – this is the normal number of chromosomes. In a cell with the diploid number of chromosomes, the chromosomes are always considered in pairs. For example, man has 23 pairs, dogs have 39 pairs and cats have 19 pairs.
- **Haploid number** – this is half the normal number of chromosomes and is seen in the germ cells. In a cell with the haploid number of chromosomes, each chromosome is unpaired.

All cells go through a cycle that results in cell division. The first phase of the **cell cycle** can be considered to be interphase (although as it is a cycle we could start anywhere). During **interphase** the cell functions normally. As it prepares to divide the cell must produce new genetic material to be put into the new cell – this occurs during the **synthesis or S phase**. The cell then rests, known as the **gap or G2 phase**, and then begins to divide by **mitosis or meiosis – called the M phase**. The two new cells produced by this division start to function normally and go into interphase, and so on.

Cells divide in one of two ways depending on their type:
- **mitosis** – the process by which **somatic cells** divide
- **meiosis** – the process by which **germ** cells divide.

Memory Jogger

Link the O of mitosis to the O in somatic cells and the E of meiosis to the E in germ cells.

- **Mitosis** – occurs during normal growth and repair and is shown by the somatic cells. Full details of the four stages of mitosis are shown in Fig. 1.2.

Before cell division occurs, the nuclear membrane dissolves and each chromosome produces an exact replica of itself, so that for a short time the cell contains twice the normal number of chromosomes. The replica and the original chromosome are then called **chromatids** and they are joined at their centres by the **centromere**. The chromatids arrange themselves along the

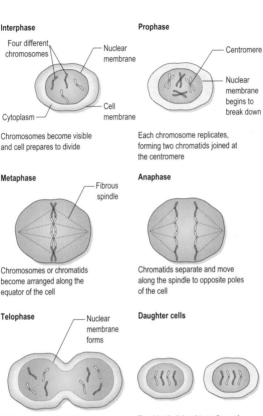

Interphase

Four different chromosomes

Nuclear membrane

Cytoplasm

Cell membrane

Chromosomes become visible and cell prepares to divide

Prophase

Centromere

Nuclear membrane begins to break down

Each chromosome replicates, forming two chromatids joined at the centromere

Metaphase

Fibrous spindle

Chromosomes or chromatids become arranged along the equator of the cell

Anaphase

Chromatids separate and move along the spindle to opposite poles of the cell

Telophase

Nuclear membrane forms

Cytoplasm begins to divide and nuclear membrane begins to reform

Daughter cells

Two identical daughter cells, each containing the diploid number of chromosomes, are produced

Figure 1.2 Mitosis – cell division in somatic cells

'equator' of the cell and then pull apart, each member of the pair moving towards one of the 'poles' of the cell. The cytoplasm of the cell splits into two and the nuclear membrane reforms around the chromosomes, forming two identical daughter cells, each containing the normal or diploid number of chromosomes.

Memory Jogger

MITOSIS occurs in SOMATIC cells and results in the formation of TWO IDENTICAL daughter cells, each containing the DIPLOID number of chromosomes. The daughter cells are identical to the parent cells.

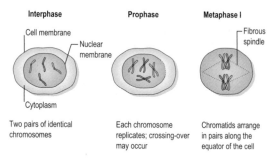

Interphase

Cell membrane
Nuclear membrane
Cytoplasm

Two pairs of identical chromosomes

Prophase

Each chromosome replicates; crossing-over may occur

Metaphase I

Fibrous spindle

Chromatids arrange in pairs along the equator of the cell

Anaphase I/Telophase I

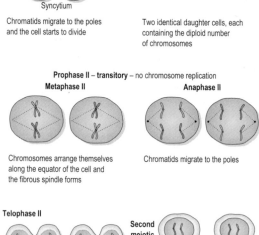

Syncytium

Chromatids migrate to the poles and the cell starts to divide

First meiotic division

Two identical daughter cells, each containing the diploid number of chromosomes

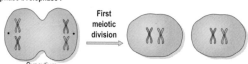

Prophase II – transitory – no chromosome replication

Metaphase II

Chromosomes arrange themselves along the equator of the cell and the fibrous spindle forms

Anaphase II

Chromatids migrate to the poles

Telophase II

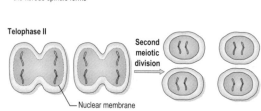

Nuclear membrane

Each cell divides and the nuclear membrane begins to reform

Second meiotic division

Four identical cells, each containing the haploid number of chromosomes. These cells are *not* identical to the parent cell

Figure 1.3 Meiosis – cell division in germ cells

Memory Jogger

The stages of MITOSIS are interphase, prophase, metaphase, anaphase, telophase. Remember the word IPMAT to help you learn the order of the stages.

- **Meiosis** – the form of cell division occurring in the germ cells – the ova in the ovary and the spermatozoa in the testes. Fig. 1.3 shows details of the stages of meiosis.

At first the chromosomes replicate and the cell divides exactly as in mitosis. This is the **first meiotic division**, which results in two identical daughter cells. The chromatids then separate from each other and the cells divide again, producing four cells, each containing half the normal number, i.e. the haploid number, of chromosomes. This is the **second meiotic division**.

At fertilisation, the haploid number of chromosomes in the nucleus of the spermatozoon combines with the haploid number in the ovum to restore the diploid number, within what is now referred to as the **zygote**. The zygote then divides by mitosis to form the embryo.

Memory Jogger

MEIOSIS occurs in the GERM cells and results in the formation of FOUR IDENTICAL daughter cells, each containing the HAPLOID number of chromosomes. The daughter cells are NOT identical to the parent cells.

Memory Jogger

The stages of MEIOSIS are interphase, prophase, metaphase I, anaphase I, telophase I, prophase II, metaphase II, anaphase II, telophase II. Think of the words IPMAT/ProMAT to help you learn the order.

MULTIPLE CHOICE

Now use these multiple choice questions to test your understanding of this chapter.

1. The study of classification is known as:

a. anatomy ○

b. taxonomy ○

c. binomial system ○

d. breeding. ○

2. Rabbits are classified as members of which order?

a. Artiodactyla ○
b. Rodentia ○
c. Carnivora ○
d. Lagomorpha. ○

3. The word 'rostral' describes structures that are:

a. towards the upper surface of the body ○
b. close to the tail ○
c. towards the nose ○
d. on the undersurface of the fore paw. ○

4. Which of the following cells divide by meiosis?

a. muscle ○
b. ovum ○
c. somatic cells ○
d. skin. ○

5. The result of cell division by meiosis is:

a. four identical daughter cells, each containing the haploid number of chromosomes ○
b. two non-identical daughter cells containing the haploid number of chromosomes ○
c. four daughter cells that are identical to the parent cells and contain the diploid number of chromosomes ○
d. two identical daughter cells that are identical to the parent cells and contain the diploid number of chromosomes. ○

6. The sequence of events during mitosis is:

a. anaphase, metaphase, telophase, prophase, interphase ○
b. interphase, prophase, telophase, metaphase, anaphase ○
c. interphase, prophase, metaphase, anaphase, telophase ○
d. telophase, metaphase, prophase, anaphase, interphase. ○

THE ANSWERS ARE:

1 b, 2 d, 3 c, 4 b, 5 a, 6 c.

2
The Body Layout

The layout of the body is easy to sort out and understand once you realise that it and all its seemingly complicated systems consist of only **four types of tissue**. These are arranged into the **organs** that make up the **body systems**, which lie within the **three principal body cavities**. Filling up all the remaining spaces in the body and lying between the cells of the tissues, around the organs and even inside the cells are **two types of body fluid**, which are described as filling **two fluid compartments**.

So you only have to remember:
- four tissue types
- three body cavities
- two fluid types in two compartments.

BASIC TISSUE TYPES

A tissue is a collection of cells and their products in which one type of cell predominates, e.g. muscle tissue and nervous tissue. These tissues are visible to the naked eye but the details are often distinguishable only under the microscope.

Every type of tissue is made up of three main components:
- **Cells** – the largest proportion of cells will be of one type, which may give the name to the tissue. For example, muscle cells form muscle tissue and fat cells form fatty or adipose tissue.
- **Intercellular products** – these are produced by the cells and lie between them.
- **Fluid** – this bathes the cells or flows between them in specialised channels.

There are four types of tissue:
- epithelial tissue
- connective tissue
- muscle tissue
- nervous tissue.

Table 2.1 Examples of where the basic tissue types can be found

Tissue type	Example
Epithelium	
Simple squamous	Blood vessels (known as endothelium), capillaries, lymphatics, lining the body cavities – pleura, peritoneum, lung alveoli
Simple cuboidal	Renal nephrons
Simple columnar	Gastrointestinal tract
Ciliated columnar	Respiratory tract
Stratified	Epidermis, oesophagus
Stratified keratinised	Claws, hooves and horns
Transitional	Ureters, bladder, urethra
Connective tissue	
Loose connective	Between organs. Beneath the dermis it occurs as the hypodermis, which connects the skin to the underlying tissues around blood vessels
Adipose or fat	Beneath the skin, behind the eye, around the kidney and in the footpads
Dense or fibrous connective	Dermis of the skin, capsules of joints, kidney, lymph nodes, ligaments, tendons and aponeuroses, muscle sheaths around skeletal muscle, scar tissue
Yellow elastic	Walls of blood vessels
Hyaline cartilage	Articular surface of joints, rings of the trachea and bronchi, larynx, nose, distal end of the ribs. Forms the skeletal model in the embryo before it becomes ossified
Fibrocartilage	Intervertebral discs, articular menisci in the stifle and temporo-mandibular joints, surrounding the glenoid fossa of the shoulder joint and the acetabulum of the hip joint
Elastic cartilage	Ear pinna, epiglottis
Compact bone	Cortex of all bones
Spongy or cancellous bone	Inside long, short and flat bones
Muscle tissue	
Smooth	Walls of blood vessels and within the visceral body systems, e.g. gastrointestinal, respiratory and urinogenital systems, inner ring of the bladder and anal sphincters
Skeletal	Attached to the skeleton; outer ring of the bladder and anal sphincters
Cardiac	Heart
Nervous tissue	Brain, spinal cord, peripheral and cranial nerves

Table 2.1 shows examples of the sites where these tissues can be found.

EPITHELIAL TISSUE

Epithelial tissue covers the entire outside of the body, and inside the body it lines all the body cavities and all the tubes of the body, e.g. blood vessels, small intestine and respiratory passages.

FUNCTION

The function of epithelial tissue is to:

- **Protect** – this is the most important function and prevents the underlying structures from being damaged by mechanical or chemical factors.
- **Absorb** – seen in some areas, such as within the small intestine, where the products of digestion are absorbed into the bloodstream.
- **Secrete** – seen in some areas, such as within the small intestine, where cells are able to secrete digestive juices, and within the renal nephrons, where cells secrete materials from the bloodstream into the glomerular filtrate.

STRUCTURE

Epithelial tissue consists of individual epithelial cells supported by a thin basement membrane which attaches them to the underlying tissue.

Epithelial tissues (Table 2.1) may be classified by the thickness of the layer and by the dimensions of the cells:

1. **Thickness of the layer**
- **Simple epithelium** – consists of a single layer of cells, e.g. cells lining the blood vessels.
- **Stratified or compound epithelium** – two or more cells thick, providing better protection. In order to increase the degree of protection the layers of the cells may contain a protein called keratin – the epithelium is described as being **keratinised**. Keratinised stratified epithelium is very tough, resistant to chemical damage and bacterial invasion, and is found in claws, hooves and horns.

2. **Dimensions of the cells**

- **Squamous epithelium** – the height of the individual cells is small, creating a flattened effect. Found lining blood vessels.
- **Cuboidal epithelium** – the height of the cells is equal to their width, so that the cells are almost cuboidal. Found lining the renal nephrons.
- **Columnar epithelium** – the height of the cells is greater than the width, so that each one is column-shaped. Found lining the intestinal tract.

Some epithelial tissues may show additional functional modifications:

- **Transitional epithelium** – a form of stratified epithelium which is capable of stretching to many times its natural size. Found lining the bladder, which expands when filling with urine.
- **Ciliated epithelium** – individual cells have small hair-like structures or **cilia** protruding from their free edges. Ciliated columnar epithelium is found lining the respiratory tract, where the cilia create a wave-like motion to waft foreign particles, e.g. dust, up the tract to the pharynx, where the cough reflex propels them out of the mouth.
- **Mucous membrane** – this covers most of the internal surfaces of the body. Specialised **goblet cells** in the epithelium secrete a sticky viscous liquid known as **mucus**, which lubricates the surface and traps foreign particles, preventing them from damaging the underlying tissue.
- **Glandular tissue** – all glands in the body are derived from epithelial tissue. They may be:
    - **Unicellular** – single cells within the epithelium, e.g. goblet cells.
    - **Multicellular** – collections of cells lying deeper in the underlying tissue. They may be:
        - **Exocrine glands** – connected to the surface by means of a **duct** through which their secretions, which may be mucoid (sticky), serous (watery) or mixed, reach their target area. A **simple** exocrine gland has an unbranched duct, e.g. sebaceous and digestive glands, while a **compound** gland has a branched

duct, e.g. mammary glands.

- **Endocrine glands** – these are **ductless** glands. Their secretions, known as **hormones**, reach their target organ via the bloodstream, e.g. thyroid and pituitary glands.
- **Mixed glands** – these have both exocrine and endocrine functions, e.g. pancreas.

CONNECTIVE TISSUE

Connective tissue is widely distributed around the body and takes many forms (Table 2.1). In order of increasing density, the connective tissues are:

- blood
- haemopoietic tissue
- loose connective tissue
- dense connective tissue
- cartilage
- bone.

All the forms of connective tissue have two components in common:

- **Intercellular matrix** – also called a **ground substance**. This may be fluid (blood), gelatinous (bone marrow) or hard (bone). If there are fibres in the matrix, it is described as **fibrous connective tissue**; the greater the proportion of fibres, the denser the connective tissue. If there are no fibres, the tissue is described as **amorphous** (without shape).
- **Associated cells** – these are distributed between the fibres and within the matrix. The cells are named according to the type of connective tissue.

The proportion of matrix in relation to the proportion of the cells determines the name and function of the tissue.

- **Blood – red blood cells (erythrocytes)** and a variety of **white blood cells (leucocytes)** suspended in a liquid matrix or **plasma** (see Chapter 6). Blood is responsible for the transport of materials around the body and plays a part in maintaining the body in a state of equilibrium or homeostasis.

- **Haemopoietic tissue** – primordial stem cells of all the types of blood cells suspended within a jelly-like matrix. This tissue forms the bone marrow within the long bones and is responsible for **haemopoiesis** – the formation of all the cellular elements of the blood.

- **Loose connective tissue** – also called **areolar** (meaning spaces) tissue. Lies between the organs and connects and supports them. It consists of a loose network of **collagen fibres** with high tensile strength and **elastic fibres**, which stretch. Distributed among the fibres are various cells, including **fibroblasts** to produce collagen, **fat cells** to provide insulation and store energy, and other cells, such as **macrophages** and **mast cells**, which are involved in the protective inflammatory response.

  - **Adipose tissue** or 'fat' is normally found in areas such as just below the skin, but it occurs in larger quantities in obese animals. It is similar to loose connective tissue but contains more fat cells, which provide insulation and protection.

- **Dense connective tissue** – also known as **fibrous connective tissue** as it contains a high proportion of collagen fibres, which have immense strength. If the fibres are arranged in parallel bundles, as seen in tendons and ligaments, it is called **regular dense connective tissue**. If the fibres form an interwoven network, as seen in the protective capsule around the kidney, it is called **irregular dense connective tissue**. The associated cells are fewer in number and are trapped in spaces between the fibres.

  - **Yellow elastic tissue** is similar to dense connective tissue but contains a higher proportion of elastic fibres, which are able to regain their shape after being stretched. It is often mixed with other tissue in sites where elasticity is needed.

- **Cartilage** – this tissue is rigid yet flexible, has high tensile strength and can bear weight. Relatively few **chondrocytes** or cartilage-forming cells are trapped within a dense network of collagen and elastic fibres and a tough gel matrix. Surrounding the cartilage is a fibrous layer or **perichondrium**, containing more numerous chondrocytes and less matrix. The perichondrium provides the blood supply to the underlying cartilage, which does not contain blood vessels. There are three types of cartilage:
  - **Hyaline** – has a clear bluish appearance. The chondrocytes tend to be arranged in parallel columns. This is the most common type and forms, for example, the articular cartilage of joints. The articular surface is not covered in perichondrium.
  - **Fibrocartilage** – contains an increased number of collagen fibres arranged in parallel bundles, which creates a tissue of increased rigidity and strength.
  - **Elastic cartilage** – contains a high proportion of elastic fibres, which enables the cartilage to spring back into shape.

- **Bone** – **osteoblasts** or bone-forming cells produce a substance called **osteoid**, which later becomes calcified to become hard bone. The cells, now known as **osteocytes**, are trapped in spaces known as **lacunae**. The osteocytes are no longer able to grow, but they communicate with each other by cytoplasmic threads inside narrow channels known as **canaliculi**. These are arranged in closely packed three-dimensional concentric circles known as **Haversian systems**. Other cells, known as **osteoclasts**, are able to remodel the bone, so that bony tissue is a constantly changing tissue. All bone is covered in **periosteum** – a fibrous outer connective tissue membrane.

There are two types of bone:
- **Compact bone** – forms the outer layer or cortex of all bones and consists of densely packed Haversian systems.
- **Spongy or cancellous bone** – spicules of bone called **trabeculae**, forming a network within the ends of long bones and the core of short and flat bones. Spaces between the trabeculae are filled with bone marrow.

MUSCLE TISSUE

The function of muscle tissue is to bring about **movement**. There are three types of muscle, which are distinguished by their structure and the way in which they are controlled by the nervous system.

- **Smooth muscle** – found lining the walls of all the visceral body systems (Table 2.1) and within the blood vessels. It also forms the inner ring of the sphincters of the bladder and anus. Its movements are controlled by the autonomic nervous system and are unconscious or involuntary.

  Each cell:
  - is spindle-shaped
  - has a central nucleus
  - is non-striated (or non-striped).

- **Striated or skeletal muscle** – found attached to the bones of the skeleton and forming the outer ring of the sphincters of the bladder and anus. It is under conscious or voluntary control.

  Each cell or **muscle fibre**:
  - is long, cylindrical and unbranched (Fig. 2.1).
  - has several nuclei, which lie towards the periphery.
  - is striated – the central part of the fibre is filled with thread-like **myofibrils**, which are the contractile elements of the muscle. The myofibrils lie parallel to each other and each consists of two contractile proteins, **actin** and **myosin**, which give the myofibril a striped or striated appearance that is visible under a microscope.
  - is surrounded by a cell membrane known as the **sarcolemma** and filled with cytoplasm known as **sarcoplasm**. This contains the organelles, such as the numerous **mitochondria** needed to provide the energy necessary for muscle contraction.

The muscle fibres are bound together in parallel by connective tissue into bundles or **fascicles**. Groups of fascicles are then bound together within a **sheath** of connective tissue to

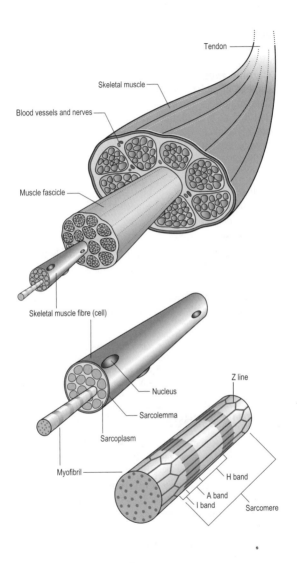

Figure 2.1 Structure of skeletal muscle

form a large skeletal muscle. The connective tissue running through the muscle carries blood capillaries and nerve fibres and eventually emerges to join with the periosteum of the bone to form a **tendon**, which attaches the muscle to the bone.

- **Cardiac muscle** – found only within the heart walls and capable of prolonged rhythmic contraction throughout life. Cardiac muscle has an inherent contractility, which means that it is able to contract at a constant rate without nervous stimulation. Control is involuntary via the autonomic nervous system, which alters the inherent rate in response to the changing needs of the body.

Each cell:
- is short, cylindrical and branched
- has a central nucleus
- is striated
- is linked to the other cells by **intercalated discs**, which facilitate rapid nerve transmission across the tissue.

Memory Jogger

To help you decide whether the muscle tissue in a particular structure is smooth or striated, consider whether you have to think consciously to make an action happen. For example, you do not have to make your blood vessels dilate or your food pass down your intestine, so the walls of these structures contain involuntarily controlled smooth muscle. In contrast, you have to decide to move your legs if you want to walk or your fingers to pick something up, so the muscles you use are made of voluntarily controlled striated muscle.

NERVOUS TISSUE

The main cell type in nervous tissue is the **neuron** and its function is to transmit nerve impulses from one area to another. Each neuron consists of:
- a **cell body** containing a **nucleus**
- several short nerve fibres called **dendrons** (thicker) or **dendrites** (thinner), through which nerve impulses enter the cell
- one long nerve fibre, called the **axon**, along which impulses are carried away from the cell.

The diameter of nerve fibres is very small – usually a few micrometres – but their length varies from a few millimetres to as much as a metre.

Many axons are covered with a **myelin sheath,** which gives the nerve fibre a whitish appearance – it is described as being **myelinated**. Myelin is a lipoprotein secreted by **Schwann cells**, which are wrapped around the axon like a Swiss roll. Between the Schwann cells are gaps known as the **nodes of Ranvier**. The function of myelin is to increase the rate of nerve transmission along the nerve fibre. Non-myelinated nerve fibres are less common but may be found within the grey matter of the brain and spinal cord, and in the retina of the eye.

Neurons in the body occur in different shapes:
- **Multipolar** – many dendrons and dendrites and one axon.
- **Pseudounipolar** – one dendron and one axon, which appear to leave the cell body from the same site. In fact they are twisted together as they leave the cell body and then separate at some distance from the cell body.
- **Bipolar** – one dendron and one axon, which leave from separate sites on the cell body.

NERVE IMPULSE TRANSMISSION

The axon of each neuron terminates in a button-like structure called a **synapse**. A synapse between an axon and a muscle fibre is called a **neuromuscular junction**. Each cell body receives many synapses from other neurons, each of which has a small effect. Their combined effect ensures the transmission of the impulse down the next axon. All nerve pathways are made up of neurons and synapses and ultimately end in a neuromuscular junction to stimulate movement of muscle tissue. The whitish structures identified by the naked eye as nerves are made up of large numbers of nerve fibres and synapses.

The nerve impulse passing along an axon is transmitted to the next cell body or to a muscle fibre by means of chemical transmitters. These transmitters, the most common of which is **acetyl choline**, are found within vesicles inside the synapse. As the nerve impulse travels along the axon the vesicles drift towards the junction between the axon and the cell body and cross the gap, initiating a nerve impulse on the other side. This process requires the presence of **calcium ions**.

THE BODY CAVITIES

The body is divided into three cavities (Fig. 2.2) in which lie the viscera or the visceral organs:

- **The thoracic cavity**, formed by the:

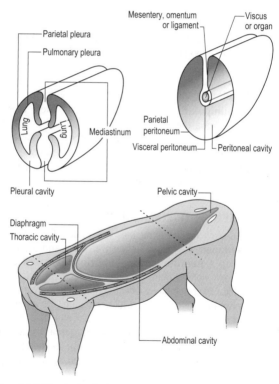

Figure 2.2 Sections to show body cavities and serous cavities schematically

- cranial thoracic aperture, made by the first pair of ribs, the first thoracic vertebrae and the manubrium
- diaphragm
- sternum
- ventral surfaces of the thoracic vertebrae
- paired ribs, forming a bony cage.
- **The abdominal cavity**, formed by the:
  - diaphragm
  - cranial pelvic aperture
  - abdominal muscles
  - diaphragm and lumbar vertebrae
  - dorsolateral, lateral and ventral muscles of the abdominal wall.
- **The pelvic cavity**, formed by the:
  - cranial and caudal pelvic apertures
  - sacrum and the first few coccygeal vertebrae
  - pubis and ischium
  - sacrotuberal ligament and associated muscles.

The thoracic and abdominal body cavities are lined by a continuous layer of squamous epithelium, which also covers the organs within it. The epithelial cells secrete a small amount of watery or **serous fluid** and the lining membranes are described as **serous membranes** surrounding the **serous cavities**. The serous fluid acts as a lubricant between the serous membranes, reducing friction as the organs move against each other. It is important to remember that a small volume of fluid is all that is found within the body cavities – the organs found within the body cavities are wrapped in the serous membrane and therefore lie outside their respective serous cavity (Fig. 2.2).

The serous membrane lining each cavity is named according to the cavity and the organ it covers:

- **Thoracic cavity** – here the membrane is called the **pleura** and it forms the right and left **pleural cavities** (Fig. 2.2). The space between them is the **mediastinum**, which contains most of the thoracic organs and their related nerves and blood vessels. The lungs, most of the left and right bronchi and their associated nerves and blood vessels push laterally out from the mediastinum, taking their covering of pleura and reducing the size of their respective pleural cavities.

- The pleura covering the lungs is the **pulmonary (or visceral) pleura**.
- The remaining pleura is the **parietal pleura**, which is subdivided into the:
  - **mediastinal pleura** – lining the mediastinum
  - **costal pleura** – lining the ribs
  - **diaphragmatic pleura** – lining the diaphragm.

The pleural cavity between the pulmonary and parietal pleurae is almost non-existent and contains only a thin film of serous or pleural fluid.

- **Abdominal cavity** – here it is called the **peritoneum** and forms the **peritoneal cavity**. This continues into the more cranial part of the **pelvic cavity**. Every organ within the abdomen is covered in the peritoneum, which originates from the dorsal wall of the cavity and is referred to as the **visceral peritoneum**. The peritoneum lining the walls of the abdominal cavity and the cranial pelvic cavity is the **parietal peritoneum**.

Most of the abdominal organs are suspended within the cavity by two layers of peritoneum, between which is a small amount of connective tissue (Fig. 2.3). These suspensory structures, known as **mesenteries**, carry fine nerve fibres and blood capillaries to and from the organs. The mesenteries are named according to the organ involved.

For example:
- The **omentum** covers the stomach – the greater omentum is attached to the greater curvature and the lesser omentum is attached to the lesser curvature.
- The **mesoduodenum** covers the **duodenum.**
- The **mesocolon** covers the **colon.**
- The **mesometrium** covers the **uterus.**

All these structures are part of one continuous layer of visceral peritoneum (Fig. 2.3).

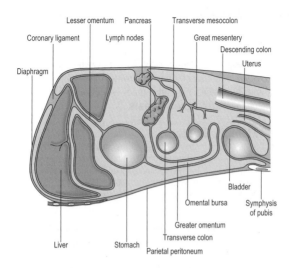

Figure 2.3 Cross-section through the abdominal cavity to show the arrangement of the peritoneum

Some organs maintain their attachment to the abdominal body wall and, although covered in a layer of parietal peritoneum, are not suspended within the cavity. They are described as being **retroperitoneal**. The peritoneal cavity is almost entirely filled by the peritoneum-covered organs and their attachments, leaving room for only a small volume of lubricating serous or **peritoneal fluid**.

- **Pelvic cavity** – there is no physical division between the abdominal and pelvic cavities, and the **peritoneum** extends into the cranial part of the pelvic cavity. Organs within the cavity are not covered with peritoneum unless they extend over the pelvic brim into the abdominal cavity, e.g. the bladder when filling, the uterus when pregnant, and the cranial part of the rectum suspended by the mesorectum. The remainder of the cavity is completely filled with connective tissue, muscles and ligaments.

BODY FLUIDS

About 60–70% of the adult body weight is made up of water, although younger animals may contain up to 75% water and older animals may contain only 55–60% water. Its function is to maintain a constant internal environment within which the metabolic processes can take place effectively. This is one of the mechanisms of **homeostasis**.

Memory Jogger
Homeostasis is the way in which the internal environment of the body is kept in a state of equilibrium so that all the body processes can work effectively. It involves osmoregulation, thermoregulation, respiration, buffers within the blood, and excretion. Maintenance of homeostasis depends on information being sent to the brain from the nervous and endocrine systems.

The body water and its dissolved contents, commonly described as body fluid, is distributed between two main fluid compartments:

- **Intracellular fluid** – represents 40% of body weight, or 66% or two-thirds of total body water.
- **Extracellular fluid** – represents 20% of body weight, or 33% or one-third of total body water.

Dissolved within the water are:

- **Organic** or carbon-based materials, such as fats, proteins and carbohydrates.
- **Inorganic** materials, such as sodium, potassium, magnesium and calcium. These exist as charged particles or ions, which are described as electrolytes or salts.

Memory Jogger
An electrolyte is a substance that breaks up into ions when dissolved in water.
An ion is a charged particle.
A cation is a positively charged particle, written as e.g. Na+ (sodium) or K+ (potassium).
An anion is a negatively charged particle, written as e.g. Cl– (chloride) or HCO_3– (bicarbonate).

Intracellular fluid (ICF) is found within the cells and can be subdivided into the fluid found:

- in the blood cells
- in all other cells.

The **main cation** of ICF is potassium (K+), although sodium (Na+) and magnesium (Mg2+) are present in lower concentrations.

The **main anion** of ICF is phosphate, with lower concentrations of bicarbonate (HCO_3-) and chloride (Cl-).

ICF also contains **proteins**.

Extracellular fluid (ECF) flows around and between the cells. It can be subdivided into three compartments:
- **Blood plasma** – surrounds the blood cells and is carried around the body by the circulatory system. Represents 5% of body weight or 0.1% of total body water.
- **Interstitial fluid** – lies between the cells but is outside the circulatory system. Represents 15% of body weight or 3% of total body water.
- **Transcellular fluid** – formed by active secretory mechanisms in the body, e.g. synovial fluid, digestive juices and cerebrospinal fluid. Its volume is always changing but on average it represents 1% of body weight or 0.02% of total body water.

The **main cation** of ECF is sodium (Na+), with lower concentrations of potassium (K+) calcium (Ca2+) and magnesium (Mg2+).

The **anions** within ECF are chloride (Cl-), bicarbonate (HCO_3-) and phosphate.

Protein is not normally present in interstitial fluid but is present in plasma. The main **plasma proteins** are:
- **globulin** – involved in the immune response
- **fibrinogen and prothrombin** – involved in blood clotting
- **albumin** – needed to maintain circulating blood volume and blood pressure.

ACID–BASE BALANCE
In order for the body to function effectively, the body fluids must be maintained at a constant pH of between 7.35 and 7.45. If

the fluid contains a high level of hydrogen (H+) ions it becomes acidic, i.e. the pH is low; if it contains a low level of H+ ions it becomes alkaline, i.e. the pH is high. In either case, several homeostatic processes will be activated to bring the pH back to normal. These processes are:

- **Actions of buffers** in the blood, e.g. haemoglobin, bicarbonate, phosphate and plasma proteins. Buffers are able to take up H+ ions in an acid environment or give up H+ ions in an alkaline environment in order to keep the pH within normal limits. They compensate for small changes in the pH.

- **Respiration** – excess carbon dioxide in the blood creates an acid pH. This stimulates the expiratory centre in the brain. The excess carbon dioxide is expired and the pH returns to normal.

- **Urine formation by the kidneys** – the distal convoluted tubule of each renal nephron secretes or resorbs H+ ions into or from the urine under the control of the hormone aldosterone (see Chapter 9).

Memory Jogger

The pH scale is a measure of the hydrogen (H+) ion concentration in a solution.

· When the level of H+ ions is high the solution is acid and the pH will be between 7 and 1.

· When the level of H+ ions is low the solution is alkaline and the pH will be between 7 and 14.

· Neutral pH is 7.

FLUID DYNAMICS

Fluid is constantly moving into and out of the body and flowing around and between the fluid compartments.

1. Water is taken into the body in food and drink, and in a normal healthy dog or cat water leaves the body in:

- **faeces** – 10–20 ml/kg body weight per day
- **urine** – 20 ml/kg body weight per day – may be called **'sensible' water loss**
- **sweat and respiration** – 20 ml/kg body weight per day – may be called **'insensible' or 'inevitable' water loss.**

Thus, a healthy animal needs to drink **50–60 ml/kg body weight per day** of fluid to compensate for this loss. Fluid may also be lost in disease conditions such as diarrhoea, haemorrhage and severe burns. Where fluid loss exceeds fluid intake the animal becomes dehydrated, and if it is to recover, the fluid must be replaced.

2. Water also flows between the body compartments within the body. This is controlled by the **osmotic pressure** and the **volume** of the ECF – mainly the plasma – and the ICF.

Memory Jogger

Osmotic pressure – the pressure needed to prevent osmosis from occurring. It depends on the number of particles of both ions and undissolved molecules in a solution.

Osmosis – the passage of water from a weaker to a stronger solution across a semipermeable membrane.

Osmotic pressure and osmosis are dependent on:

- **Electrolyte concentration** – if the osmotic pressure of the plasma is too high, e.g. the concentration of sodium ions is too strong, then fluid will flow into the plasma by osmosis until there are equal concentrations on either side of the blood capillary walls. If the osmotic concentration is too low fluid will flow out of the plasma into the extracellular spaces.
- **Plasma proteins** – these are large molecules that under normal circumstances are unable to pass between the endothelial (epithelial) cells lining the blood capillaries. They draw water from the extracellular fluid into the plasma by osmosis, so maintaining the volume of the blood and the pressure it exerts on the wall of the blood vessels – blood pressure. In inflamed areas, as a result of histamine release, the junctions between the endothelial cells widen and the plasma protein molecules escape into the extracellular fluid, drawing more fluid from the plasma.

The osmotic pressure or tonicity of a fluid is described relative to plasma and is an important consideration when selecting fluids for fluid replacement therapy:

- **Isotonic** – the osmotic pressure of the fluid is the same as that of plasma. Most fluids given parenterally are isotonic and there is no movement of fluid between compartments.

- **Hypotonic** – the osmotic pressure of the fluid is lower than that of plasma. If the fluid is added to the ECF, water moves into the cells, resulting in cell rupture and consequent cell death.
- **Hypertonic** – the osmotic pressure of the fluid is higher than that of plasma. If the fluid is added to the ECF, water is drawn out of the cells and they become dehydrated.

The replacement fluid must be as close as possible, in terms of electrolyte content and osmotic pressure, to the fluid that has been lost.

BODY SYSTEMS

Within the body the tissues are combined to form complex organs which are arranged into systems linked by a common function. Table 2.2 shows the body systems and their functions. Those systems that lie within one of the body cavities are described as the **visceral systems** or the 'viscera'.

Memory Jogger
· A tissue is a collection of cells and their products in which one type of cell predominates, e.g. muscle tissue, nervous tissue.
· An organ is a collection of different tissues that work together to form a particular tissue, e.g. the heart is made of muscle, connective, nervous and epithelial tissues.
· A system is a collection of parts, structures, organs and tissues that are linked by their contribution to a common function, e.g. the respiratory system.

MULTIPLE CHOICE

Now use these multiple choice questions to test your understanding of this chapter.

1. Which of the following is not a function of epithelial tissue?

a. absorption   ○

b. protection   ○

c. secretion   ○

d. movement.   ○

Table 2.2 Systems of the animal body

Name of system	Principal organs	Function
Skeletal system	The bones of the skeleton, linked by joints	Supports the body and provides a framework for the attachment of muscles
Muscular system	The muscles of the head, limbs, trunk	Brings about movement and locomotion
Nervous system	Brain, spinal cord, nerves, special sense organs	Receives information from the external and internal environment, analyses it and initiates the appropriate rapid response
*Blood vascular system	Heart, blood and lymphatic vessels, blood	Carries oxygen and nutrients to the tissues and carries waste materials produced by the tissues to a site where they can be excreted
*Respiratory system	Nasal cavities, trachea, bronchi and lung tissue	Takes in oxygen and excretes carbon dioxide
*Digestive system	Mouth, oesophagus, stomach, small intestine, large intestine	Digests food and absorbs the products of digestion
*Urinary system	Kidneys, bladder, urethra	Excretes nitrogenous waste and maintains the balance of water and electrolytes
*Reproductive system	Female – ovaries and uterus Male – testes and penis	Produces the next generation of offspring
Endocrine system	Pituitary, thyroid, parathyroids, pancreas, ovary, testis, adrenal glands	Controls the functions of the body by chemical messengers (hormones), which produce a slow but long-lasting response
Integument	Skin, hair, claws, footpads	Provides a protective covering for the body

*Denotes a visceral system.

2. Which type of epithelial tissue is found lining the bladder?

a. simple stratified ○
b. transitional ○
c. ciliated columnar ○
d. keratinised. ○

3. Which type of muscle is found within the walls of the blood vessels?

a. smooth ○
b. skeletal ○
c. cardiac ○
d. striped. ○

4. The main cation of intracellular fluid is:

a. magnesium ○
b. sodium ○
c. calcium ○
d. potassium. ○

5. In order to compensate for normal daily fluid loss a healthy animal needs to drink:

a. 20–30 ml/kg body weight ○
b. 30–40 ml/kg body weight ○
c. 50–60 ml/kg body weight ○
d. 70–80 ml/kg body weight. ○

6. If the osmotic pressure of a fluid is lower than that of plasma it is described as being:

a. hypotonic ○
b. isotonic ○
c. hypertonic ○
d. barotonic. ○

THE ANSWERS ARE:

1 d, 2 b, 3 a, 4 d, 5 c, 6 a.

3
The Locomotor System

The locomotor system enables an animal to move from place to place to find food, new territories, sexual partners or escape from predators. The system can be considered as two separate parts that work together to bring about locomotion. They are:

- **the skeletal system**
- **the muscular system.**

THE SKELETAL SYSTEM

The skeletal system consists of the bones forming the **skeleton** and the **joints**, which link the bones together. The skeleton forms the rigid framework of the body and consists mainly of bone and cartilage.

Memory Jogger

Bone consists of osteocytes trapped within a calcified matrix and arranged in concentric lamellae known as Haversian systems. The outer surface is covered in periosteum. There are two types of bone – compact and spongy or cancellous bone.

Cartilage consists of chondrocytes in a dense network of collagen and elastic fibres and a tough gel matrix. The outer surface of all cartilage, except that forming the articular surface of joints, is covered in perichondrium. There are three types of cartilage – hyaline, fibrous and elastic.

Refer to Chapter 2.

BONE DEVELOPMENT AND GROWTH

Within the developing embryo, bone tissue forms and grows in one of two ways depending on the type of bone:

- **Intramembranous ossification** – flat bones including many of the bones of the skull develop in this way. New bone forms between two layers of periosteum.

- **Endochondral ossification** – all limb bones develop in this way. A hyaline cartilage model forms and becomes ossified or changed to bone. One or two centres of ossification appear and bony tissue gradually spreads within the cartilage until the final bone takes shape. A thin plate of cartilage may be trapped at the ends of the bone and it is from here that the bone is able to grow in length – this is the **epiphyseal plate**, which closes over when the animal reaches its final size.

SKELETON

The **functions** of the skeleton are to:
1. support the body
2. provide leverage for locomotion
3. protect the soft tissues within the body
4. act as a storage organ for calcium and phosphorus.

Finding your way around the skeleton (Fig. 3.1)
There are over 200 bones in the skeleton. To enable us to study and to describe them accurately they can be divided into several categories. Descriptive names are given to the various lumps, bumps and holes that cover them.

Classification of bones

- **Long bones** – long and more or less cylindrical. Each end is called the **head** – either distal or proximal; the middle is the **shaft**. The outer layer of bone or **cortex** is made of compact bone while the centre or **medullary cavity** is hollow. The ends of the bone are filled with spongy bone and haemopoietic tissue. Examples: humerus, femur, radius, metatarsals.
- **Short bones** – may be many-sided but have similar dimensions of height, width and depth. Consist of outer compact bone filled with spongy bone. No medullary cavity. Examples: carpal bones.
- **Flat bones** – two layers of compact bone separated by a thin layer of spongy bone. Examples: ribs, scapula and some skull bones.
- **Irregular bones** – unpaired, lie in the midline of the body and have an asymmetrical shape. Consist of outer compact and inner spongy bone. Example: vertebrae.
- **Sesamoid bones** – sesame-seed shaped bones associated with joints and often set within tendon tissue. They change the direction of pull of a tendon as it runs over the joint. Examples: patella, fabellae.
- **Pneumatic bones** – contain air spaces known as sinuses. Examples: maxilla, frontal.

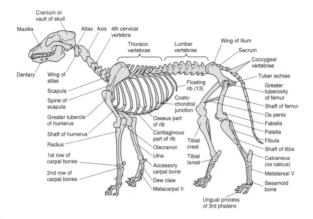

Figure 3.1 The skeleton of the dog

Descriptive terminology

In order to provide accurate information about the sites of disease or injury, the bony landmarks are given scientific names. The best way to learn these is to explore the skeleton and relate it to the living animal.

- **Foramen** – a hole within a bone (plural foramina) through which blood vessels and nerves pass. Some larger structures, such as the spinal cord, may also pass through foramina.
- **Projection** – a part of a bone that projects outwards may be called a **dens, ridge, crest, condyle, trochanter, tuberosity, tubercle or process.**
- **Depression** – a part of a bone that goes inwards may be called a **fossa or fovea, cavity or groove.**

The skeleton (Fig. 3.1) can be divided into three parts:

- **Axial skeleton** – runs from the head to the tip of the tail, forming the axis of the animal. It consists of the skull, vertebral column and rib cage.
- **Appendicular skeleton** – consists of the appendages: the pectoral and pelvic limbs and the pectoral and pelvic girdles, which attach them to the body.
- **Splanchnic skeleton** – bones which lie within soft tissues and are not attached to the main skeleton.

AXIAL SKELETON

Skull

The **functions** of the skull are to:

1. protect the brain
2. support and provide attachment for the muscles of mastication, swallowing, vocalisation and facial expression
3. provide a bony channel through which inspired air can enter the body.

The skull consists of the **cranium**, a box-shaped structure that houses the brain and is attached to the two **nasal chambers**. The lower jaw, consisting of the **right and left mandibles** and the **hyoid apparatus**, is suspended from the cranium.

The bones of the skull (Fig. 3.2) are joined together by fibrous joints known as **sutures**. These do not allow much movement but permit a small amount of growth in young animals and may become replaced by bone during the ageing process.

The **frontal** and **maxillary** bones contain air-filled cavities or **sinuses**, which connect with the nasal chambers (see Chapter 7).

The **nasal chambers** are two tubes formed by the **incisive** and **maxillary bones** (Fig. 3.2). The narrow roof is formed by the **nasal bone** and the floor by the **palatine bone**. The chambers are separated by a cartilaginous **nasal septum** and are filled with delicate scrolls of bone – the **conchae or ethmoturbinates** (see Chapter 7).

The **hyoid apparatus** is a collection of delicate bones forming a swing-like structure (Fig. 3.2). The tongue is attached to the rostral side and the larynx to the caudal side. The whole apparatus is suspended from the **petrous temporal** bone.

The **right and left mandibles** (Fig. 3.2) are joined in the midline by the **mandibular symphysis**. Each mandible consists of the horizontal **body** and vertical **ramus**. Each ramus articulates with the rest of the skull at the **temporomandibular joint**.

Cranium and nasal chambers

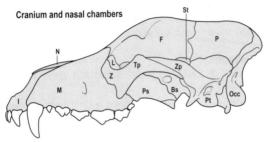

I – Incisive bone
M – Maxilla
N – Nasal
L – Lachrymal
Z – Zygomatic arch
Tp – Temporal process of zygomatic arch

Zp – Zygomatic process
P – Parietal
F – Frontal
Occ – Occipital
Pt – Petrous temporal

St – Squamous temporal
Ps – Presphenoid
Bs – Basisphenoid

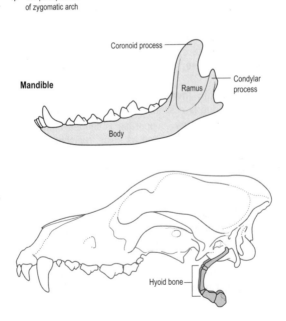

Mandible

Coronoid process

Condylar process

Ramus

Body

Hyoid bone

Figure 3.2 Parts of the canine skull

The skull is perforated by numerous **foramina**, through which blood vessels and nerves pass into and out of the cranial cavity. The largest of these is the **foramen magnum** in the occipital bone, through which the spinal cord leaves the base of the brain and travels down the vertebral canal.

Skull shape

- The skull of the cat is apple-shaped and varies very little between breeds.
- The shape of the dog skull shows great variation between breeds, achieved by centuries of selective breeding from the original wolf type. It may be described as:

    dolichocephalic – long thin nose and lower jaw, e.g. borzoi, greyhound, Afghan hound

    mesaticephalic – average-shaped head, e.g. beagle, spaniel

    brachycephalic – short, pushed-in nose as a result of shortening of the nasal chambers, hard palate and lower jaws, e.g. pug, boxer, bulldog.

- The upper jaw (incisive and maxillary bones) and the lower jaw (mandibles) should be of equal length to produce an effective bite. Sometimes the jaws are of unequal length:

    prognathic jaw – upper jaw is longer than the lower jaw – the dog is described as being 'undershot'

    epignathic jaw – upper jaw is shorter than the lower jaw – the dog is described as being 'overshot'.

Vertebral column

The **functions** of the vertebral column are to:

1. protect the spinal cord
2. provide a stiff but flexible rod to support the body
3. provide attachment for the rib cage and muscles, which protect the internal organs.

The vertebral column consists of a chain of irregular unpaired bones or **vertebrae** running down the midline of the body from the base of the skull to the tip of the tail.

Table 3.1 Regional variations of the vertebral column

Region of vertebral column	Number of vertebrae	Identifying features
Cervical	7 – all mammals have the same number regardless of the size of the neck	C1 – the atlas – consists only of a pair of flattened transverse processes or wings. Articulates with the occipital condyles of the skull and allows a nodding movement of the skull C2 – the axis – has a long body with a cranial projection – the dens – which articulates with the caudal side of C1 allowing rotating movement of the skull C3 to C7 – follow the standard design and get progressively smaller
Thoracic	13	All have tall spinous processes whose height progressively decreases, and short bodies. Two depressions or fovea articulate with the proximal end of the ribs – the costal fovea forms a synovial joint with the head of the rib; the transverse fovea forms a synovial joint with the tubercle of the rib
Lumbar	7	Have large transverse processes angled cranioventrally, and large bodies
Sacral	3	Vertebra are fused together to form the wedge-shaped sacrum. Forms the sacroiliac joint with the wing of the ilium of the pelvic girdle
Coccygeal or caudal	Number depends on the length of the tail	The most proximal follow the basic shape but they get progressively smaller and simpler towards the tip of the tail

Vertebral shape

The shape of each vertebra is based on a common plan (Fig. 3.3) and consists of:

- A cylindrical **body** – the cranial surface is convex while the caudal surface is concave, enabling the vertebrae to interlock to form a flexible rod. They are separated by fibro-cartilaginous **intervertebral discs**, which act as shock-absorbers during locomotion. The dorsal surface of the body is flattened and forms the floor of the **vertebral foramen**.

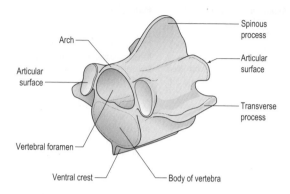

Spinous process

Articular surface

Arch

Articular surface

Transverse process

Vertebral foramen

Ventral crest

Body of vertebra

Figure 3.3 Basic shape of a vertebra

- **A vertebral arch** – arises from either side of the body to complete the vertebral foramen. When the vertebrae are linked together, the vertebral foramina form the **vertebral canal**, through which the spinal cord runs.
- **A spinous process** – arises from the dorsal surface of the vertebral arch. Its height varies according to the region of the vertebral column (Table 3.1). Provides a surface for the attachment of epaxial spinal muscles and ligaments (see The muscular system).
- **A pair of transverse processes** – project laterally and vary in size and shape according to the region. Provide a surface for the attachment of the spinal muscles and ligaments and they separate these muscles into the epaxial and hypaxial muscle groups (see The Muscular System, p. 51).

On each vertebra there is a pair of **cranial articular processes** and **caudal articular processes**. Each one articulates with the process on the preceding or following vertebra by means of a synovial joint. The vertebra is also penetrated by numerous foramina, through which blood vessels and nerves travel. The most significant one is formed by a notch on the caudal and cranial surfaces (Fig. 3.3). When the vertebrae come together they form the **intervertebral foramina** on either side of the vertebral column. The spinal nerves leave the spinal cord through these foramina.

The vertebral column is divided into regions according to its position in the body. Each region contains a characteristic number of vertebrae, each with certain identifying features, which differentiate them from the common plan (Table 3.1).

Rib cage

The **functions** of the rib cage are to:

1. form the thoracic cavity
2. protect the soft tissues within the thoracic cavity
3. enable respiration to take place.

The rib cage is suspended from the vertebral column and is formed by the ribs, the sternum and the thoracic vertebrae (Table 3.1).

- The **ribs** consist of 13 pairs of elongated, flat bones forming the walls of the cage. Each pair corresponds to a thoracic vertebra and consists of a dorsal bony part and a ventral cartilaginous extremity, known as the **costal cartilage**. The junction between the two parts is the **costochondral junction**. The dorsal end forms two synovial joints between the **head** of the rib and the **costal fovea** of the vertebra and between the **tuberculum** of the rib and the **transverse process** of the vertebra.

To complete the rib cage, each pair of ribs forms a synovial joint with the sternum. However, some ribs do not articulate directly:

- Ribs 1–8 articulate with the sternum – known as **true or sternal** ribs.
- Ribs 9–12 touch the costal cartilage of the rib in front – known as **asternal** ribs (Fig. 3.1).
- Rib 13 is short and the ventral end is free – this is the **floating** rib.

The caudal boundary of the rib cage formed by this arrangement of ribs is known as the **costal arch**. The intercostal spaces between the individual ribs are filled with the two layers of intercostal muscle necessary for respiration (see The Muscular System, p. 51).

- The **sternum** forms the floor of the thoracic cavity and is made up of eight bones or **sternebrae** linked by cartilaginous joints. The most cranial sternebra or **manubrium** is larger than the rest, while the most caudal is flattened and forms the **xiphoid process**. It is extended by a thin caudally directed projection known as the **xiphoid cartilage**.

APPENDICULAR SKELETON

The pectoral or thoracic limb (Fig. 3.1)

This consists of the pectoral girdle, the forelimb and the forefoot.

- **Pectoral girdle** – there is no bony attachment between the limb and the trunk; the connection is made entirely by muscles running from the scapula and humerus to the head, neck and thorax. During locomotion the scapula moves slightly over the wall of the thorax. The pectoral girdle comprises:

    • **Clavicle** – a thin spicule of unconnected bone lying within the muscle running between the forelimb and the head and neck. Only in the cat.

    • **Scapula** – a large triangular flat bone applied to the wall of the thorax between ribs 1 and 4. On the lateral side it has an obvious **spine**, to which are attached the supraspinatus, infraspinatus, trapezius and deltoid muscles. The distal end forms the shallow **glenoid cavity**, into which the head of the humerus fits to form the **shoulder joint** (Table 3.2).

- **Forelimb** – consists of the following bones:

    • **Humerus** – the largest bone in the forelimb. This is a long bone with a slight twist in the region of the mid-shaft. At the proximal end the **head** forms the shoulder joint with the distal end of the scapula. The point of the shoulder is formed by the **greater tubercle**. The distal end is formed by a pair of rounded processes, the **lateral and medial condyles**, between which is the **trochlea**. In the dog, the **supratrochlear foramen** lies above the trochlea. The **olecranon** of the ulna fits into the trochlea to form the **elbow joint**.

Table 3.2 The major synovial joints of the body

Joint	Type	Description	Movement
Shoulder	Ball and socket	Formed by the head of the humerus and the glenoid cavity of the distal scapula. Joint is held in place by well-developed muscles	Flexion and extension. Small amount of rotational movement in the dog and cat
Elbow	Hinge	Formed by the distal humerus and the proximal ends of the radius and ulna. On the proximal ulna the point of the elbow is formed by the olecranon, which is extended as the beak-shaped anconeal process. Below this on the cranial border is the trochlear notch, the distal end of which forms the medial and lateral coronoid processes. The beak of the anconeal process fits between the condyles of the humerus, which provides stability. All held together by strong medial and lateral ligaments	Flexion and extension
Hip	Ball and socket	Formed by the head of the femur and the acetabulum of the pelvic girdle. A fibrous connective tissue capsule runs around the rim of the acetabulum to deepen the cavity. Within the joint the round or teres ligament attaches the head of the femur to the acetabular fossa. Joint is held in place by well-developed muscles	Flexion and extension. Small amount of rotational movement in the dog and cat
Stifle	Hinge	Formed by the distal femur and proximal tibia. The condyles of the distal femur are divided by the trochlear groove in which the patella runs. The proximal tibia is flattened with a projection known as the tibial crest on its dorsal surface. The tendon of the quadriceps femoris muscle runs over the patella on the dorsal surface of the stifle joint and inserts on the tibial crest. On the back of the joint is a pair of fabellae. Within the joint are the posterior and anterior cruciate ligaments, which stabilise the joint and a pair of cartilaginous menisci	Flexion and extension

- **Radius** – the most medial of the two bones forming the lower forelimb. It is the main weight-bearer. The proximal end articulates with the condyles of the humerus; the distal end articulates with the proximal row of the bones of the carpus.
- **Ulna** – with the radius this forms the lower forelimb, and is larger and longer than the radius. On the proximal end the point of the elbow is formed by the **olecranon**, which is extended as the beak-shaped **anconeal process**. Below this, on the cranial border, is the **trochlear notch**, the distal end of which forms the **medial and lateral coronoid processes**. These landmarks are all involved in the formation of the elbow joint (Table 3.2).
- **Carpus** – consists of seven short bones arranged in two rows. The top row, of three bones, articulates with the distal ends of the radius and ulna. Most movement occurs in this joint. The lower row, of four bones, articulates with the metacarpals.
- **Forefoot** – each foot contains five **metacarpals**, numbered 1–5. The most medial is number 1 and, as it is related to the short dew claw, is reduced in size. The proximal end of each metacarpal is flattened and articulates with the distal row of carpal bones. The distal end is transversely cylindrical and articulates with its respective proximal phalanx (plural phalanges). Metacarpals 2–5 have a pair of tiny sesamoid bones or **fabellae** on the **palmar** or undersurface of each metacarpophalangeal joint. Each metacarpal bone articulates with a **digit**. Each digit consists of a **proximal phalanx**, a **medial phalanx** and a **distal phalanx**. These are similar in shape to the metacarpals but are shorter. Digit 1 is short and known as the **dew claw**. As this does not touch the ground it bears no weight. Each distal phalanx terminates in a claw-shaped **ungual process**, which is covered by the **claw**.

Pelvic limb

This consists of the pelvic girdle, the hind limb and hind foot (Fig. 3.1).

- **Pelvic girdle** – consists of two halves, each formed from three flat bones:
  - **Ilium** – most of this is vertical and forms the cartilaginous **sacroiliac joint** with the sacrum. The **wing** of the

ilium is the most cranial part of the pelvic girdle and can be palpated easily.

- **Ischium** – forms the floor and the most caudal part of the pelvic girdle. The **ischial arch** can be palpated in the perineal area of the animal.

- **Pubis** – lies between the other two bones and forms the cranial part of the floor of the pelvic girdle.

Memory Jogger
To remember the position of each bone within the pelvic girdle – you Sit on your iSchium – so this is the most caudal of the bones, leaving the ilium as the most cranial of the three. The pubis fits in between the two.

The two halves of the pelvic girdle meet in the centre and are joined at the **pubic symphysis**. On each side of this and lying in the floor of the pelvic girdle is a large hole, the **obturator foramen**. The three bones meet to form the articular cavity of the hip joint – the **acetabulum**, into which the head of the femur fits. The centre of the acetabulum has no articular cartilage and forms the **acetabular fossa**. The **round or teres ligament** runs from this point to attach to the head of the femur to stabilise the hip joint (Table 3.2).

- **Hind limb** – consists of the following bones:
  - **Femur** – a long bone that forms the hip joint with the acetabulum of the pelvic girdle. The proximal end consists of the **head**, to which the **round or teres ligament** attaches, and a narrowed area known as the **neck**. Close to this are two roughened areas for the attachment of muscles: the **greater and lesser trochanters**. The point of the hip is the greater trochanter. The distal end of the femur is formed by a pair of rounded processes, the **lateral and medial condyles**, between which is a **trochlear groove**. The distal end of the femur articulates with the proximal end of the tibia and the patella, forming the **stifle joint** (Table 3.2).
  - **Fibula** – the finer of the two bones that form the lower hind limb. It is separate from the tibia and bears very little weight. On the distal end is the **lateral malleolus**, which can be palpated on the lateral side of the tibiotarsal or hock joint.
  - **Tibia** – the larger of the two bones of the lower limb.

It lies medial to the fibula. The proximal end is flattened and forms part of the **stifle joint** with the femur (Table 3.2). On the cranial surface is the **tibial crest or tibial tuberosity**, which is the point of insertion of the quadriceps femoris muscle. The distal end articulates with the **talus** (one of the tarsal bones) and has a deep groove within it to conform to the trochlea of the talus. The **medial malleolus** can be palpated on the medial aspect of the tibiotarsal joint.

- **Tarsus** - also called the hock. Consists of seven short bones arranged in two rows. In the proximal row, the **talus or astragalus** articulates with the tibia and allows most of the movement. The **calcaneus** is closely applied to the talus and has a large process called the **os calcis**, to which the Achilles tendon attaches. The distal row contains four bones, which articulate with the metatarsals of the hind paw. Lying between the two rows is the **central tarsal** bone.
- **Hind foot** - consists of metatarsal bones and phalanges arranged in a pattern similar to that of the forefoot. The under surface of the hind foot is known as the plantar surface.

Memory Jogger

To differentiate between the greater tubercle of the humerus and the greater trochanter of the femur, remember that horses canter using their hind legs so the trochanter is on the femur of the hind limb; this leaves the tubercle on the humerus of the forelimb.

SPLANCHNIC SKELETON

This consists of bony structures that lie within soft tissues and so provide added strength. In the dog and the cat the only bone is the **os penis**, which lies within the cavernous erectile tissue of the penis. In the cat it lies ventral to the urethra, which passes through it on its way to the external surface, and in the dog it lies dorsal to the urethra.

The function of the os penis is to aid introduction of the penis into the female's vagina during the early part of the mating process (see Chapter 10).

JOINTS

A joint is an area where two or more pieces of bone or cartilage are connected. May also be called an **articulation** or an **arthrosis**. Joints may be strengthened by the addition of bands of dense connective tissue that link bone to bone and are called **ligaments**.

Joints may be classified by their:

1. **Degree of movement**
   - **A synarthrosis** (plural synarthroses) is a fibrous or cartilaginous joint that allows very little movement, such as a suture or symphysis.
   - **A amphiarthrosis** (plural amphiarthroses) is a fibrous or cartilaginous joint that allows a moderate amount of movement.
   - **A syntosis** (plural syntoses) is a joint that has become fused by bone. Usually a result of the ageing process.
   - **A diarthrosis** (plural diarthroses) is a synovial joint that allows free movement.

2. **Type of action**
   - **Hinge** – the shapes of the bones involved in the joint allow movement in one plane only. Examples: elbow, stifle.
   - **Ball and socket** – a rounded head fits into a cup-shaped socket, allowing a wide range of movement, though this may be limited in quadrupeds. Examples: shoulder and hip joints.
   - **Pivot** – one bone rotates around a peg formed by another bone. Examples: atlanto-axial joint between C1 and C2.
   - **Gliding** – bones with flattened surfaces glide over each other, such as within the carpus and tarsus.

3. **Structure and connecting medium** – this is the internationally recognised system for classifying joints.
   - **Fibrous joints** – connected by dense fibrous connective tissue and allow very little movement (synarthroses); e.g. sutures of the head.
   - **Cartilaginous joints** – connected by cartilage. May be found joining opposite sides of the body; e.g. mandibular and pubic symphyses. These allow very little movement

(synarthroses). The joints between the bodies of the vertebrae are also cartilaginous and allow moderate movement (amphiarthroses).

- **Synovial joints** – contain a pale yellow viscous fluid
  called **synovial fluid**. These joints allow free movement
  (diarthroses).

All synovial joints comprise two or more bones, which are:
- covered in an articular surface of **hyaline cartilage** that
  is not covered in perichondrium
- connected by a **joint capsule** of dense fibrous connective tissue that is continuous with the perichondrium of the
  bone; it may be further strengthened by fibrous or collateral ligaments running in the capsular tissue.

The joint capsule is lined with a **synovial membrane**, which
secretes synovial fluid to lubricate the joint and act as a shock
absorber.

Within the cavity of some synovial joints there may be:
- One or more **fibrocartilaginous articular discs or
  menisci**, which effectively divide the cavity into two. There
  are two menisci in the stifle joint and one in the temporomandibular joint of the skull.
- **Ligaments** – these provide extra stability to the joint.
  Within the hip joint there is the **teres or round ligament** and within the stifle there is a pair of **cruciate
  ligaments**.

For descriptions of the major joints of the body see Table 3.2.

DEFINITIONS OF MOVEMENTS

When the muscles that are attached to the bones of the skele-
ton contract they shorten, pulling the bones close together. The
resulting movements can be defined thus:
- **Flexion** – the angle between two bones is reduced.
- **Extension** – the angle between two bones is increased.
- **Gliding** – the articular surface of one bone slides over
  another.
- **Rotation** – the bone rotates around its long axis.
- **Circumduction** – the distal end of a bone describes a

circle or a segment of one, e.g. when the undersurface of the paw is rotated upwards.

- **Pronation** – the plantar/palmar surface of the hind or fore paw is turned upwards.
- **Supination** – the plantar/palmar surface of the hind or fore paw is turned downwards.

The following terms refer to movement of the whole limb:
- **Abduction** – limb is moved away from the midline.
- **Adduction** – limb is moved towards the midline.
- **Protraction** – limb is moved cranially or forwards.
- **Retraction** – limb is moved back towards the body.

THE MUSCULAR SYSTEM

The muscular system consists of the skeletal muscles, which are attached to the bones of the skeleton. They are made of striated muscle fibres and are under voluntary or conscious control. The main function of skeletal muscle is to bring about movement of the parts of the body. Where the limbs are involved, movements are coordinated by the nervous system to bring about locomotion.

Memory Jogger
· Each striated muscle cell or fibre is long, cylindrical and unbranched and contains several nuclei, which lie towards the edge of the cell. The centre is filled with bundles of parallel thread-like myofibrils. These are made of two contractile proteins, actin and myosin, which give the fibres a striated appearance when seen under the microscope.
· The muscle fibres are bound together in parallel by connective tissue into fascicles. Groups of fascicles are then bound within a sheath of connective tissue to form a large skeletal muscle.
Refer to Chapter 2.

SKELETAL MUSCLE STRUCTURE

Every skeletal muscle comprises:
- **An origin** – the point of attachment to the bone. Connective tissue within the muscle bundles extends as a **tendon**, which merges with the periosteum of the bone connecting the muscle to the bone. May also be known as the **head** of the muscle; some muscles have several heads, such as the biceps (meaning two heads). The origin moves the least during muscle contraction.

- **An insertion** – similar to the origin in structure but at the opposite end of the muscle.
- **A belly** – the swollen central part of the muscle.

Not all skeletal muscles conform to this classic shape. Some are arranged as sheets of muscle attached by flattened bands of dense connective tissue known as **aponeuroses**.

Where a muscle or tendon runs over a bony prominence or where two muscles rub against each other, a synovial sac known as a **bursa** (plural bursae) may develop to cushion the area and reduce the effect of friction. In some cases a bursa may develop in an abnormal position; this is known as an **adventitial bursa**.

In certain parts of the body, such as the lower limbs, the elongated tendons extending from muscle bellies higher up the limb are protected from rubbing by elongated forms of bursae, which wrap around the tendon and are known as **tendon or synovial sheaths**.

Every skeletal muscle is attached to at least two points, which can be described according to the site of attachment:
- **Extrinsic muscles** – one end is attached to a point on a limb, for example, while the other end is attached to a point away from the limb, such as the trunk. Extrinsic muscles are responsible for moving the whole structure.
- **Intrinsic muscles** – both the origin and the insertion are on the same structure, e.g. the limb. They are responsible for moving parts of the structure.

MUSCLES OF SPECIFIC AREAS OF THE BODY

This section describes some of the most important skeletal muscles. In this book these are not always specifically named. If you wish to learn more, it is suggested that you read a more detailed textbook from the list of further reading at the end of the book.

Muscles of the head

1. **Muscles of facial expression** - intrinsic muscles that are responsible for moving the lips, nostrils, eyelids and ears. The eyeball is moved by a separate group of muscles that are extrinsic to the eyeball (i.e. attached to the sclera and to the orbit of the skull) but intrinsic to the head.

2. **Muscles of mastication** - intrinsic muscles responsible for the chewing action essential for breaking up food in the mouth.

- **Masseter** - runs from the lateral surface of the mandible to the ventral surface of the zygomatic arch and overlies the angle of the jaw. Closes the jaw.

- **Temporal** - lies within the temporal fossa of the skull and is attached to the coronoid process of the mandible. Closes the jaw.

- **Digastricus** - runs from the occipital bone of the skull and attaches to the angle of the mandible on its ventral surface. Opens the jaw.

3. **Muscles of the tongue** - comprise both extrinsic muscles, which run from the tongue to the pharynx, and intrinsic muscles, which enable the tongue to curl, flatten and move from side to side. These delicate movements are essential for eating, grooming and vocalisation.

4. **Muscles of the pharynx, larynx and soft palate** - involved in swallowing, vocalisation and respiration.

Muscles of the trunk

1. **Muscles of the vertebral column** - the muscles are divided into:

- **Epaxial muscles** – these lie dorsal to the vertebral column and attach to the pelvis, sacrum, ribs and individual vertebrae. Some of the muscles run long distances along the spine while some run over only two or three vertebrae. There is a great deal of intertwining, which makes it difficult to identify individual muscles.

  Their **function** is to:
  - support the spine
  - assist movement as the animal runs
  - support the weight of the head, neck and tail
  - allow a certain amount of rotation by the individual vertebrae.

- **Hypaxial muscles** – finer muscles that lie ventral to the vertebrae. Their function is to keep the thoracolumbar region of the spine dorsally concave and the cervical region ventrally concave.

2. **Muscles of the thorax** – these form an inner layer consisting of the intercostal muscles and an outer or superficial layer.

- **Intercostal muscles** – these muscles are used in respiration and lie within the intercostal spaces.

  - **External intercostals** – attach to the caudal border of each rib and run in a caudoventral direction to the cranial border of the rib in front. Involved in inspiration.

  - **Internal intercostals** – attach to the cranial border of each rib and run cranioventrally to the caudal border of the rib behind. Assist in expiration.

- **Diaphragm** – lies within the body cavity, separating it into thoracic and abdominal cavities. It is caudally concave, consists of a central tendon surrounded by a ring of striated muscle, and is suspended from the lumbar vertebrae by two muscular crura (singular, crus). To enable some structures to pass between the two body cavities, it is perforated by three holes:

  - **Postcaval foramen** – carries the caudal vena cava on its way to the heart.

  - **Oesophageal hiatus** – carries the oesophagus on its way to join the stomach.

  - **Aortic hiatus** – carries the aorta from the heart to

the rest of the body, the azygous vein and the thoracic duct, which transports lymph from the hind end of the body to the heart.

- **Superficial muscles** – three muscles form an outer protective layer over the ribs and intercostal muscles.

  - **Trapezius** – runs from C3 to C7 to the spine of the scapula, forming a triangular muscle. It draws the forelimb forward and raises the forelimb.

  - **Latissimus dorsi** – lies behind the shoulder and attaches to the lateral aspect of the thorax. It draws the trunk forward, abducts the forelimb and depresses the spine.

  - **Brachiocephalicus** – runs from the cervical vertebrae to the midshaft of the humerus. It draws the limb forward and flexes the neck.

Muscles of the abdomen

The abdominal muscles are:

- **the external abdominal oblique**
- **the internal abdominal oblique**
- **the transversus abdominis**.

These form each side of the abdominal body wall, enclosing and protecting the soft tissues within the abdominal cavity. The muscle fibres run in all directions, which gives great strength. They all end in aponeuroses, which join together in the midline as the **linea alba**.

- **Rectus abdominis** – this forms two large bands of muscle, one on each side of and overlying the linea alba. It runs along the ventral abdomen from the first rib to the prepubic tendon cranial to the pubic symphysis. It supports the abdomen and flexes the lumbar spine.

Within the area of the groin or inguinal area is a slit in the aponeurosis of the external abdominal oblique. This is the **inguinal ring**, which allows structures such as the spermatic cord to pass from the abdominal cavity to the testes in the scrotum and blood vessels to pass to the mammary glands and the external genitalia (see Chapter 10).

Table 3.3 The major muscles of the forelimb

Muscle	Location	Action
Trapezius	Originates on C3–C7 and inserts on the spine of the scapula	Raises the foreleg and draws the leg forwards
Brachiocephalicus	Originates on the cervical spine and inserts on the midshaft of the humerus	Draws the forelimb forwards, abducts the forelimb and depresses the spine
Deltoid	Originates on the spine of the scapula and inserts on the proximal humerus	Flexes the shoulder
Supraspinatus	Originates in the supraspinous fossa of the scapula and inserts on the greater tuberosity of the humerus	Extends and stabilises the shoulder
Infraspinatus	Originates in the infraspinous fossa of the scapula and inserts on the lesser tuberosity of the humerus	Flexes, extends and stabilises the shoulder
Triceps brachii	Has 4 heads which run from the scapula and humerus and all insert on the olecranon of the elbow	Extends the elbow
Biceps brachii	Originates on the scapular tuberosity and inserts on the proximal ends of the radius and ulna	Extends the shoulder and flexes the elbow
Brachialis	Originates below the head of the humerus and inserts on the olecranon	Flexes the elbow
2 carpal flexors – flexor carpi radialis and flexor carpi ulnaris	Originate from the distal humerus, proximal radius and proximal ulna, run behind the carpus and insert on the palmar side of the carpus and digits	Flexes the carpus
2 digital flexors – superficial digital flexor and deep digital flexor	Originate from the distal humerus, proximal radius and proximal ulna, run behind the carpus and insert on the palmar side of the digits	Flex the digits
Extensor carpi radialis	Originates on the distal humerus, runs in front of the carpus and inserts on the proximal ends of metacarpals 2 and 3	Flexes the elbow and extends the carpus
2 digital extensors – common digital extensor and the lateral digital extensor	Originate on the distal humerus, proximal radius and proximal ulna, run in front of the carpus and foot to insert on the dorsal surface of the digits	Extend the carpus and digits

Muscles of the forelimb (Table 3.3)
The muscles responsible for flexing and extending the joints of the distal parts of the forelimb are all located around the upper part of the limb. Tendons leading from the muscle bellies run down the limb and insert on the bones of the lower limb and forefoot. This pattern is repeated in the hind limb.

Muscles of the hind limb (Table 3.4)

1. The **hamstring group** of muscles is responsible for providing the propulsive force of the hind limb. They are enormously enlarged in animals built for speed, such as the horse and the racing greyhound. The muscles that form the hamstring group are:
   - biceps femoris
   - semitendinosus
   - semimembranosus.

   The muscle tendons forming the **Achilles tendon** are attached to the **os calcis** of the hock and are responsible for extending the hock joint. If the Achilles tendon ruptures or is cut, the point of the hock drops down to touch the ground. The tendons involved are those of the following muscles:
   - gastrocnemius
   - biceps femoris
   - semitendinosus
   - superficial digital flexor.

2. The **adductor group** of muscles all adduct the limb or bring it in towards the midline of the body. They are the:
   - pectineus
   - adductor
   - gracilis
   - sartorius.

Table 3.4 The major muscles of the hind limb

Muscle	Location	Action
Gluteals – superficial, middle and deep	Originate on the bones of the pelvis and the femur	Extend the hind limb and provide the main propulsive force of the hind limb
Quadriceps femoris	Has 4 heads, which originate around the ilium and the proximal femur and insert on the tibial tuberosity	Flex the hip and extend the stifle
Biceps femoris (hamstring group; forms part of the Achilles tendon)	Originates from the ischium and inserts on the distal femur and the os calcis of the hock	Extends the hip and hock and flexes the stifle
Semitendinosus (hamstring group; forms part of the Achilles tendon)	Originates on the ischium and inserts on the proximal tibia and the os calcis	Extends the hip and hock and flexes the stifle
Semimembranosus (hamstring group)	Originates on the ischium and inserts on the distal femur and proximal tibia	Extends the hip and hock and flexes the stifle
Pectineus (adductor group)	Originates from the cranial part of the pubis and inserts on the medial side of the femur	Adducts the thigh
Gracilis (adductor group)	Originates on the pubic symphysis and inserts on the tibia and the calcaneus	Adducts the thigh, extends the hip, flexes the stifle and extends the hock
Adductor (adductor group)	Originates from the pubic symphysis, ischium and pubis and inserts on the medial side of the femur	Adducts the thigh and extends the hip
Sartorius (adductor group)	Originates on the pelvis, runs on the medial side of the thigh and inserts on the patella	Adducts the thigh, flexes the hip and extends the stifle
Gastrocnemius (Achilles tendon)	Originates on the medial femur and inserts on the os calcis of the hock	Extends the hock and flexes the stifle
Anterior tibialis	Originates on the proximal tibia and inserts on the lateral side of the tarsus	Flexes the hock and rotates the paw medially

Muscle	Location	Action
2 digital flexors - superficial digital flexor (part of the Achilles tendon) and deep digital flexor	Originate on the distal femur and proximal tibia and fibula, run behind the tarsus and insert on the plantar surface of the digits	Superficial digital flexor - flexes the hock, extends the stifle and flexes the digits Deep digital flexor - extends the hock and flexes the digits
2 digital extensors - long digital extensor and lateral digital extensor	Originate from the distal end of the femur and the proximal fibula, run in front of the tarsus and insert on the dorsal surface of the digits	Extends the digits

Memory Jogger

The belly of the gastrocnemius muscle forms the bulge on the caudal side of the lower hind limb and contains the popliteal lymph node. This is one of the most easily palpated lymph nodes of the body. Refer to Chapter 6.

MULTIPLE CHOICE

Now use these multiple choice questions to test your understanding of this chapter.

1. Which of the following bones is NOT part of the axial skeleton?

a. hyoid apparatus ○

b. sternum ○

c. humerus ○

d. frontal. ○

2. The skull of the borzoi dog is described as being:

a. prognathic ○

b. brachycephalic ○

c. mesaticephalic ○

d. dolichocephalic. ○

3. How many cervical vertebrae make up the neck of the dog and cat?

a. 3 ○

b. 7 ○

c. 13 ○

d. 6. ○

4. Which of the following joints comprises a pair of condyles, an olecranon, an anconeal process, a trochlear notch and the lateral and medial coronoid processes?

a. elbow ○

b. hip ○

c. stifle ○

d. hock. ○

5. A syntosis is described as being:

a. a fibrous joint that allows a moderate amount of movement ○

b. a synovial joint that allows free movement ○

c. a joint that has become fused with bone ○

d. a cartilaginous joint that allows very little movement. ○

6. Which of the following muscles is part of the hamstring group but NOT part of the Achilles tendon?

a. semitendinosus ○

b. biceps femoris ○

c. semimembranosus ○

d. superficial digital flexor. ○

THE ANSWERS ARE:

1 c, 2 d, 3 b, 4 a, 5 c, 6 c.

4

The Nervous System and the Special Senses

At first, the nervous system seems to be extremely complicated but it can be more easily understood when you realise that you have a form of nervous system in your own house. Somewhere in your house you will have a central controller for your heating system. Distributed around your house are sensors that send information about the environmental temperature to the controller, which then sends hot water along the pipes to the radiators and the house warms up or cools down. Within an animal's body are sensory receptors that gather information about the external and internal environments of the body and send it to the central nervous system. Here the information is processed and nerve impulses are sent out to structures such as muscle tissue or secretory glands, and an appropriate change is made to suit the situation. Thus, the nervous system simply consists of:

- a central nervous system – the brain and spinal cord
- a variety of receptors, including those described as the 'special senses', to gather information
- a connecting system of nerve fibres passing to and from the central nervous system.

THE NERVOUS SYSTEM

The **functions** of the nervous system are to:
1. receive information from the environment – both external and internal
2. analyse and integrate the information
3. bring about the appropriate response.

The function of the nervous system depends on the passage of nerve impulses along nerve fibres, which run to and from all parts of the body. The functional unit of the nervous system is the **neuron** and it is from this that the more complex structures of the nervous system develop.

Although the nervous system is a single well-integrated unit, for the purposes of description it can be divided into two parts:

- **Central nervous system** – consisting of the brain and spinal cord.
- **Peripheral nervous system** – consisting of all the nerves given off by the central nervous system. This can be further subdivided into:
  - cranial nerves – leaving the brain
  - spinal nerves – leaving the spinal cord
  - autonomic nervous system – made up of spinal nerves supplying the visceral organs and divided into the sympathetic and parasympathetic nervous systems.

CENTRAL NERVOUS SYSTEM (CNS)

The CNS comprises the **brain** and the **spinal cord**. Control by the CNS is **voluntary or conscious**, meaning that the animal is aware of making a movement or feeling pain.

The tissue of the CNS consists of **grey matter and white matter**, which are distinguished by their myelin content.

- **Grey matter** – consists of groups of cell bodies of the neurons and contains very little myelin. It forms a butterfly-shaped central core in the spinal cord, and in the brain it is mixed with the white matter, forming discrete islands known as **ganglia or nuclei**.
- **White matter** – consists of myelinated nerve fibres and is found around the outside of the spinal cord and in the inner layers of the brain.

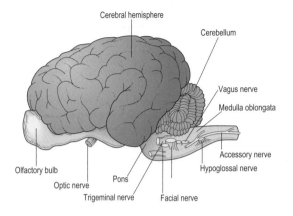

Figure 4.1 Lateral view of the canine brain

Memory Jogger
Myelin is a whitish lipoprotein produced by the Schwann cells, which surrround many nerve fibres. Its function is to insulate the fibres, facilitating rapid transmission of nerve impulses from one area to another.
Refer to Chapter 2.

The brain

The brain is a hollow convoluted organ that is housed within the cranial cavity of the skull. In its simplest form it can be considered to consist of three parts:

- forebrain
- midbrain
- hindbrain.

1. **The forebrain** – this is the largest and most obvious part of the brain (Fig. 4.1). It consists of three main parts:
- **Cerebrum or right and left cerebral hemispheres** – occupies the greater part of the forebrain and contains 90% of all the neurons in the entire nervous system. It is involved in conscious thought and comprises:
  - two cerebral hemispheres divided into distinct lobes by deep **fissures**

- the **corpus callosum**, a tract of white matter that links the two hemispheres across the midline
- an outer layer of grey matter known as the **cerebral cortex**
- a deeply folded surface – the upfolds are called **gyri** (singular gyrus) and the depressions are called **sulci** (singular sulcus).

- **Thalamus** – lies deep within the tissue of the forebrain. Its function is to process information from the sense organs and relay it to the cerebral cortex.
- **Hypothalamus** – lies below the thalamus and forms the floor of the brain. It has three vital functions:
  - links the nervous and endocrine systems by secreting a range of releasing hormones that stimulate the production of hormones from other endocrine glands (see Chapter 5)
  - assists in the control of the autonomic nervous system, affecting a range of involuntary activities, such as sweating, shivering, vasodilation and vasoconstriction
  - has a major effect in maintaining a constant environment within the body – **homeostasis**; maintains the body fluid balance, regulates body temperature and controls hunger and thirst.

Memory Jogger

Homeostasis is the way in which the internal environment of the body is kept in a state of equilibrium so that all the body processes can work effectively. It involves osmoregulation, thermoregulation, respiration, buffers within the blood, and excretion. Maintenance of homeostasis depends on information being sent to the brain from the nervous and endocrine systems.

On the ventral surface of the forebrain are:
- The **optic chiasma**, which is a crossover for fibres of the optic nerve. This ensures that information from one eye goes to both sides of the brain.
- The **pituitary gland**, which lies below the hypothalamus and secretes a wide range of hormones (see Chapter 5).
- A pair of **olfactory bulbs** forming the most rostral point of the brain. They receive olfactory nerve fibres from the mucosa lining the nasal chambers.

2. **The midbrain** is a short length of brain almost

completely overhung by the forebrain. It acts as a pathway for nerve fibres running from the fore- to the hindbrain and vice versa.

3. **The hindbrain** consists of three main parts.

- **Cerebellum** – lies on the dorsal surface, caudal to the cerebrum (Fig. 4.1). It comprises two hemispheres, each of which is covered in deep folds with an obvious division into inner white and outer grey matter. Its function is to control balance and muscular coordination.

- **Pons** – lies ventral to the cerebellum, forming a transverse bridge of nerve fibres running from one cerebellar hemisphere to the other. It contains nerve centres involved in the control of respiration.

- **Medulla oblongata** – extends from the pons to the beginning of the spinal cord as it leaves the cranial cavity (Fig. 4.1). The pons and medulla form the brainstem. It contains centres that control respiration and blood pressure.

Protection of the brain

The brain is a vital organ without which an animal cannot function normally. It is protected from damage by several different structures:

1. The bones forming the **cranial cavity** of the skull protect the soft tissues from physical damage.

2. Within the cranial cavity the brain is wrapped in several membranous layers known as **meninges**. These continue down the vertebral canal to protect the spinal cord. From the outside inwards, the meninges are the:

- **Dura mater** – a tough, fibrous connective tissue layer that is continuous with the periosteum of the bones of the cranium. In the vertebral canal there is a space between the dura mater and the periosteum of the vertebrae. This is the **epidural space**, which is filled with fat and blood capillaries.

- **Arachnoid mater** – a network of collagen fibres. Above this is the **subdural space** and below it, filled with cerebrospinal fluid, is the **subarachnoid space**.

- **Pia mater** – a delicate membrane which is closely attached to the surface of the brain, following all the gyri and sulci.

3. The brain is filled with and surrounded by **cerebro-**

spinal fluid (CSF). This clear, slightly yellow fluid, which resembles plasma without the protein content, acts as a shock absorber and provides the nervous tissue with nutrients. CSF flows in the subarachnoid space around the brain and spinal cord, and inside the brain it flows within a series of linked cavities or **ventricles**. The **ventricular system** comprises:

- The **central canal** – a narrow channel running along the centre of the spinal cord.
- The **fourth ventricle** – continuous with the central canal, which widens as it enters the hindbrain.
- The **cerebral aqueduct or aqueduct of Sylvius** – leads from the fourth ventricle and progresses as a narrow channel running through the midbrain.
- The **third ventricle** – a blind-ending cavity that lies within the forebrain and is continuous with the cerebral aqueduct. It gives off a **lateral ventricle** into each cerebral hemisphere.

Samples of CSF can be collected from the **cisterna magna** between the cerebellum and the medulla oblongata.

The spinal cord

This is a glistening white structure that runs from the medulla oblongata to the lumbar region of the vertebral column. It is entirely protected by the bony vertebral canal formed by the interlinked vertebrae. At about the seventh lumbar vertebra, the cord breaks up into a group of spinal nerves running together to form the **cauda equina**, which supplies the caudal end of the body. The spinal cord is segmented. Each segment corresponds to a vertebra and gives off a pair of **spinal nerves**, which carry nerve impulses to and from the CNS.

In cross-section the spinal cord comprises:

- A butterfly-shaped area of **grey matter** (Fig. 4.2) surrounding the **central canal**, which contains CSF and is part of the ventricular system.
- An outer area of **white matter**, which surrounds the grey matter. This consists of organised tracts of white matter, which run up towards the brain (ascending tracts) or away from the brain to the effector organs (descending tracts). Each tract has a definite origin and destination, which makes response time as short as possible.

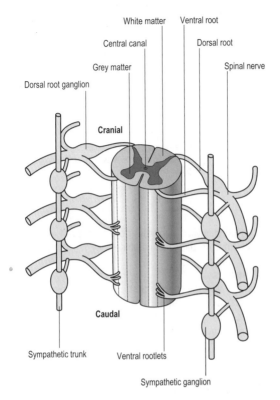

White matter   Ventral root

Central canal   Dorsal root

Grey matter   Spinal nerve

Dorsal root ganglion

Cranial

Caudal

Sympathetic trunk   Ventral rootlets

Sympathetic ganglion

Figure 4.2 Cross-section through the spinal cord

Memory Jogger
Grey matter contains non-myelinated nerve fibres and the cell bodies of the neurons, while white matter is so called because it contains nerve fibres which are wrapped in the white lipoprotein myelin. Refer back to the beginning of the chapter.

PERIPHERAL NERVOUS SYSTEM

The peripheral nervous system consists of the nerves given off by the CNS. These are the cranial nerves from the brain and the spinal nerves from the spinal cord.

Table 4.1 Classification of nerves

Type of nerve	Definition
Sensory	Carries nerve impulses towards the CNS
Motor	Carries nerve impulses away from the CNS
Mixed	Contains both sensory and motor fibres
Intercalated neuron	Lies between a sensory nerve and a motor nerve
Efferent	Carries impulses away from a structure (may be the CNS)
Afferent	Carries impulses towards a structure (may be the CNS)
Visceral	May be sensory or motor. Supplies organs within the visceral body systems, i.e. respiratory, heart, urinogenital and digestive systems
Somatic	May be sensory or motor. Supplies structures that lie in the skin or the musculoskeletal system

Nerves can be classified according to the types of organs that they supply and the direction in which they run (Table 4.1).

Cranial nerves
Cranial nerves are those nerves that emerge from the brain and leave the cranial cavity through the numerous foramina that penetrate it. They have specific names, which in many cases describe their actions, and are distinguished by Roman numerals (Table 4.2). They may be sensory, motor or mixed nerves (Table 4.1).

Memory Jogger
To remember the names of the cranial nerves you may like to invent a mnemonic, but a useful one to use is:
'**O**h, **o**h, **o**h **t**o **t**ouch **a**nd **f**ondle **v**icious **g**iraffes, **v**icunas **a**nd **h**amsters.'
This corresponds to **o**lfactory, **o**ptic, **o**culomotor, **t**rochlear, **t**rigeminal, **a**bducens, **f**acial, **v**estibulocochlear, **g**lossopharyngeal, **v**agus, **a**ccessory, **h**ypoglossal.

Spinal nerves
Each segment of the spinal cord gives off a pair of spinal nerves – one to the left and one to the right – which leave the vertebral canal by the **intervertebral foramina**, formed by the notches on the caudal and cranial edges of each vertebra (see Chapter 3).

Spinal nerves are **mixed** nerves (Table 4.1). Each nerve consists of:

Table 4.2 The cranial nerves

Number	Name	Type	Description
I	Olfactory	Sensory	Carries sense of smell or olfaction from nasal mucosa to the olfactory bulbs
II	Optic	Sensory	Carries the sensation of sight from the eyes to the cerebral hemispheres
III	Oculomotor	Motor	Supplies extrinsic muscles of the eyes
IV	Trochlear	Motor	Supplies extrinsic muscles of the eyes
V	Trigeminal	Mixed	Supplies the muscles of mastication Carries sensation from the skin around the eye and face
VI	Abducens	Motor	Supplies extrinsic muscles of the eyes
VII	Facial	Motor	Supplies the muscles of facial expression
VIII	Vestibulocochlear or auditory	Sensory	Cochlear branch carries information about hearing from the cochlea Vestibular branch carries information about balance from the semicircular canals
IX	Glossopharyngeal	Mixed	Carries sense of taste or gustation from the taste buds. Supplies the muscles of the pharynx
X	Vagus	Mixed	Carries sensation from the pharynx and larynx. Supplies muscles of the larynx, heart and smooth muscle and glands of the thoracic and abdominal viscera
XI	Accessory	Motor	Supplies muscles of the neck and shoulder
XII	Hypoglossal	Motor	Supplies muscles of the tongue

- A **dorsal root** – carries sensory nerve fibres from peripheral receptors towards the spinal cord. Close to the cord on each spinal nerve is a **dorsal root ganglion** (Fig. 4.2) containing the cell bodies of the sensory neurons.
- A **ventral root** – carries motor nerve fibres away from the spinal cord. There is no ganglion associated with this branch. All the cell bodies are found within the ventral part of the grey matter (Fig. 4.2).
- One or more **intercalated neurons** linking the sensory and motor nerves. The intercalated neurons lie within the grey matter of the cord.

The spinal nerves supply the entire musculoskeletal system. In the region of the pectoral and pelvic girdles they are thicker than anywhere else, forming the **brachial plexus** supplying the forelimb and the **lumbosacral plexus** supplying the hind limb.

Reflex arcs

A reflex arc is a fixed involuntary response to a particular stimulus and involves only the spinal nerve for that segment. Information is received by receptor cells within the skin, joints, muscles and special sense organs, and is carried to the spinal cord by sensory nerves.

Taking the **withdrawal or pedal reflex** as an example, the path of a reflex arc is as follows:

1. The web of the paw is pinched.
2. The sensation is detected by receptors in the skin and is carried by sensory nerves to the relevant segment of the spinal cord.
3. Motor nerve impulses are sent out from the spinal cord to the muscles of the limb; the muscles contract and the paw is withdrawn.

The brain is not involved in a reflex arc. However, taking the withdrawal reflex as an example, if the dog responds by biting this means that nerve impulses have also passed up the ascending tracts of white matter to the brain and pain has been consciously perceived. Nerve impulses are sent to the muscles of the jaw, and the dog bites.

Reflex arcs may be **simple or monosynaptic,** involving only one synapse within the spinal cord, or **polysynaptic**, involving at least one intercalated neuron within the cord.

Reflexes may be overridden by the brain or **conditioned**. For example, you can force yourself to hold your hand under hot water even though the muscles of your arm are trying to contract and pull your hand away. The classic example of a conditioned reflex is Pavlov's dogs – the stimulus for normal salivation in dogs was changed from the sight and smell of food to a ringing bell. Conditioned reflexes are used in toilet-training puppies and kittens.

Table 4.3 The autonomic nervous system

	Sympathetic nervous system	**Parasympathetic nervous system**
Origin of the nerve fibres	Arise from the first thoracic vertebra to the fourth or fifth lumbar vertebra	Cranial nerves III (oculomotor), VII (facial), IX (glossopharyngeal) and X (vagus) all contain fibres. Also arise from first and second sacral vertebrae
Site of ganglia containing cell bodies	Close to the dorsal body wall under the vertebral column, forming the sympathetic chain	Close to the appropriate organ or within it
Preganglionic fibres, i.e. fibres leading from the CNS to the ganglia	Short	Long
Postganglionic fibres, i.e. fibres leading from the ganglia to the organ	Long	Short
Transmitter substance at synapses within the nerve pathway	Acetylcholine	Acetylcholine
Transmitter substance at the terminal synapse in the effector organ	Noradrenaline	Acetylcholine
General effect	Prepares the body for 'fear, flight, fight'. Heart and respiratory rates increase. Blood vessels to skeletal muscles dilate. Bronchi and bronchioles dilate. Stress levels increase	Respiratory and heart rates reduce. Salivation, peristalsis and secretion of digestive juices increase. Stress levels fall

Autonomic nervous system

The autonomic nervous system is a man-made division consisting of spinal nerves from specific regions of the spinal cord. It may be considered to be a **visceral motor system** because all the nerves leave the CNS and supply the smooth muscle and glandular tissue within the viscera and the blood vessels.

The autonomic nervous system is divided into two parts, which occupy different areas of the body and have opposite effects. They are the:

- sympathetic nervous system
- parasympathetic nervous system.

Most organs have a supply of both types and control is a balancing act between the two.

Details of the two systems can be found in Table 4.3.

THE SPECIAL SENSES

To function effectively, the nervous system must receive information about the body's internal and external environments. Distributed throughout the body are several types of receptors whose function is to gather this information and pass it to the CNS. There are three types of receptor cell:

1. **Interoreceptors** – provide the CNS with information about the state of the internal environment. They include osmoreceptors, chemoreceptors and baroreceptors, which monitor parameters such as levels of oxygen and carbon dioxide in the blood, pH of the blood, and blood pressure. The information is conveyed to the brain, initiating a series of reactions to maintain the internal environment in a balanced state – known as **homeostasis**. These reactions are unconscious and are vital for the normal function of the body.

2. **Proprioceptors** – provide the CNS with information about the position of the body in relation to the external environment. They are found in muscles and joints and monitor the angle of a joint or the tension or degree of stretch in a muscle. Proprioceptors work in conjunction with the sense of balance located in the inner ear.

3. **Exteroreceptors** – provide the CNS with information about the external environment and gather the conscious sensations or **special senses** of taste, smell sight, hearing and balance. Touch is detected by specialised exteroreceptors known as **Pacinian corpuscles**, which are distributed throughout the skin. Specialised

organs have evolved to house the exteroreceptors –
these are the **special sense organs**.

TASTE – ALSO CALLED GUSTATION

The receptor organs are the **taste buds**, which are distributed
within the mucosa covering the dorsal surface of the tongue,
the epiglottis and the soft palate. They consist of **gustatory
cells**, leading from which are delicate nerve fibres that are
branches of the cranial nerves responsible for carrying the sensation of taste to the brain – the facial (VII), glossopharyngeal
(IX) and vagus (X) nerves. The gustatory cells are **chemoreceptors**, which respond to the chemicals responsible for taste.
These chemicals dissolve in the mucus covering the taste buds,
and the resulting nerve impulses are then carried to the brain,
where they are interpreted as taste.

SMELL – ALSO CALLED OLFACTION

Receptor cells lie within the **olfactory mucosa** lining the dorsocaudal part of the nasal chambers. Leading away from each
receptor cell (each of these cells is also a chemoreceptor) are
fine nerve fibres, which are branches of the **olfactory nerve (I)**.
The chemicals responsible for smell dissolve in the mucus covering the membrane and the resulting nerve impulses pass
along the olfactory nerve fibres and enter the **olfactory bulbs**
of the forebrain, where they are interpreted as smell. Gustation
and olfaction are closely allied and they often work together.

SIGHT

Photoreceptors within the retina of **the eye** (Fig. 4.3) are
adapted to respond to the stimulus of light.

- All mammals have a **pair** of eyes, which are set on the
  head in a position related to their lifestyle. For example,
  predators need **binocular vision** to accurately locate and
  catch prey, so the eyes lie on the front of the head. Prey
  species need **monocular vision**, which provides a wide field
  of view to enable them to see their predators; however,
  this type of vision is less accurate so the eyes lie high up
  on the sides of the head.
- Each eye is set in a bony protective **orbit** within the skull.

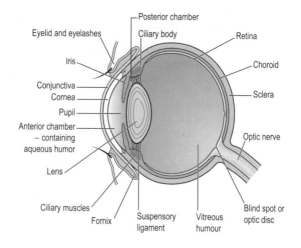

Figure 4.3 Structure of the canine and feline eye

- Each eye is further protected by an **upper and a lower eyelid**, which join at the angles of the eye; these angles are known as the **medial canthus** (close to the nose) and the **lateral canthus**. Both eyelids consist of palpebral muscles covered with an outer layer of hairy skin and lined with a continuation of the conjunctiva. On the upper eyelid is a row of **eyelashes or cilia**.
- In addition, the cat and the dog have a **third eyelid**, which is a T-shaped piece of cartilage and smooth muscle set in the medial canthus; it provides additional protection underneath the upper and lower eyelids.
- All three eyelids are supplied with glands, the most notable of which are the **Meibomian** and **lacrimal glands**. These secrete fluids to lubricate and protect the anterior part of the eye.
- Each eyeball is globe-shaped and consists of three layers (Fig. 4.3):

- **Sclera** – tough, fibrous and protective this forms the posterior two-thirds of the outer layer and the transparent **cornea** forms the front of the eye. The extrinsic muscles of the eye are inserted in the sclera. The cornea is covered with a protective layer of squamous epithelium known as the **conjunctiva**. The junction between the two is the **corneal–scleral junction** or the **limbus**.

- **Uvea** – the vascular pigmented middle layer, which consists of the:

   a. **Choroid** – forms two-thirds of the uvea. Contains blood capillaries that supply all the internal structures of the eyeball.

   b. **Tapetum lucidum** – an area of iridescent cells lying in the dorsal part of the uvea that reflect light back to the photoreceptor cells of the retina, so making better use of low light levels.

   c. **Ciliary body** – a thickened part that projects in towards the centre of the eye. Contains the ciliary muscles, which are able to change the shape of the lens.

   d. **Suspensory ligament** – this continuation of the ciliary body forms a circular support around the periphery of the lens.

   e. **Iris** – an anterior continuation of the ciliary body projecting in front of the lens. The free edge forms the **pupil**. The size of the pupil is altered by the smooth muscle fibres within the iris to control the amount of light reaching the retina.

- **Retina** – the innermost layer. Contains the photoreceptor cells, which are known as **rods** (black and white or night vision) and **cones** (colour vision). These are sandwiched between an outer layer of bipolar nerve cells and an inner layer of pigmented cells. Nerve impulses generated by the effect of light striking the photoreceptor cells pass across the retina via the overlying nerve cells and leave the eye through the **optic nerve** (Fig. 4.3).

Memory Jogger

To remember which of the photoreceptor cells is responsible for which function, make the link between **CO**NES and **CO**LOUR vision, which leaves RODS and BLACK and WHITE vision.

Within the eyeball:

- The area in front of the iris forms the **anterior chamber** and contains **aqueous humour**. The area between the iris and the lens is known as the **posterior chamber**.
- Behind the iris, the lens, suspensory ligament and ciliary body form the boundary of the jelly-like **vitreous humour** (Fig. 4.3). The function of both the aqueous and the vitreous humour is to maintain the shape of the eye and to provide nutrients for the structures within the eye.
- The **lens** is a biconvex transparent disc suspended in the midline by the suspensory ligament and ciliary body. Its function is to focus light onto the retina. The lens tissue is elastic and its shape is altered by the contraction of the ciliary muscles around it.

Perception of light – light rays from an object pass through the **cornea**, which plays a part in focusing the light onto the retina. The amount of light entering the eye is controlled by the size of the **pupil**. The light rays strike the **lens** and are focused onto the **retina** by altering the curvature of the lens. This is done by the **ciliary muscles**. Light rays pass through the layers of the retina until they hit the **photoreceptor cells**.

The photoreceptor cells are stimulated and the resulting nerve impulses pass via the **optic nerve** (II) to the brain, where they are interpreted as sight.

HEARING AND BALANCE

Receptor cells that respond to sound waves and to movement of the body are found within the inner **ear** (Fig. 4.4).

- All mammals have a **pair** of ears set high up on the head.
- Each ear is divided into three parts:

  External ear – consists of a funnel-shaped **pinna** made of cartilage and covered in hairy skin, the function of which is to guide sound waves down the ear canal. It also plays an important part in communication between animals of the same species. The cartilage of the pinna continues as the tube-shaped **external auditory meatus or ear canal**. This runs vertically down the side of the skull and then turns inwards to run horizontally into the skull. The ear

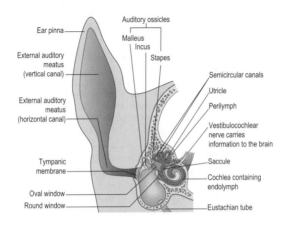

Figure 4.4 Section through the canine and feline ear

canal is lined with modified skin containing a few hair follicles and ceruminous glands, which produce a protective wax; it terminates at the **tympanic membrane or eardrum** (Fig. 4.4).

● **Middle ear** – an air-filled cavity within the tympanic bulla of the skull. It contains the **auditory ossicles**: the **malleus** (hammer), **incus** (anvil) and **stapes** (stirrup). These form a flexible chain of bones linked by synovial joints lying across the cavity – the malleus is in contact with the tympanic membrane while the stapes is in contact with the oval window of the inner ear. Opening into the cavity of the middle ear is the **Eustachian tube**, leading from the pharynx. Its function is to maintain equal pressure on either side of the tympanic membrane, so that it remains flexible and functional.

● **Inner ear** – consists of a **bony labyrinth** (Fig. 4.4) carved out of the petrous temporal bone of the skull, which conforms to the shape of the membranous labyrinth lying within it. The bony labyrinth is linked to the middle ear by the **round window** and the **oval window** and is filled with a fluid known as **perilymph**. The **membranous labyrinth** is a system of interconnecting tubes filled with a fluid known as **endolymph**.

Memory Jogger

To learn where the perilymph and endolymph lie within the inner ear, remember that the prefix 'peri-' means 'surrounding' or 'around' (e.g. perimeter, periphery) and the prefix 'endo-' means 'inside'. Thus, perilymph surrounds the membranous labyrinth while the endolymph lies inside the membranous labyrinth.

The inner ear has three parts, each with a different function:

1. **Semicircular canals** – three canals, each one describing two-thirds of a circle and set in a plane that is approximately at right angles to the other two. Within the canals are sensory receptor cells, leading from which are minute nerve fibres, which are branches of the vestibular branch of the vestibulocochlear nerve or cranial nerve VIII.

2. **Vestibule** – consists of two sac-like structures, the **utricle and saccule**, which connect the semicircular canals to the third part, the cochlea. Inside the vestibule are more sensory receptor cells, which also have nerve fibres of cranial nerve VIII leading from them.

Perception of movement – the receptor cells in the semicircular canals are responsible for monitoring an animal's movements while those in the vestibule monitor the position of an animal when it is standing still. As the animal moves, the endolymph surrounding the receptor cells moves small hair-like processes projecting from them, and the resulting nerve impulses are conveyed to the brain by the vestibulocochlear nerve. Within the brain the information is interpreted and coordinated by the cerebellum. Nerve impulses are sent to the skeletal muscles to bring about the muscle contractions required to keep the animal balanced.

3. **Cochlea** – this is a blind-ending, ventrally spiralled tube rather like a snail's shell (Fig. 4.4). It conforms exactly to the cochlear part of the bony labyrinth and is filled with endolymph. Within the cochlea are groups of sensory receptor cells forming the **organ of Corti**. Leading from the base of each cell is a minute nerve fibre which is part of the cochlear branch of the vestibulocochlear nerve.

Perception of sound – sound travels through the air as waves or vibrations, which are picked up by the funnel-shaped pinna and travel down the external auditory meatus to the tympanic membrane. The waves cause the tympanic membrane to vibrate, which in turn causes the auditory ossicles in contact with them to vibrate. The vibrations are transmitted across the middle ear to the oval window, which leads into the inner ear. Here, the vibrations cause the perilymph in the bony labyrinth to move, causing the endolymph in the cochlea to vibrate. The receptor cells within the organ of Corti are stimulated by these vibrations and the resulting nerve impulses are transmitted by the vestibulocochlear nerve to the brain, where they are interpreted as sound.

MULTIPLE CHOICE

Now use these multiple choice questions to test your understanding of this chapter.

1. Which of the following parts of the brain is responsible for the control of balance?

a. pons ○
b. cerebral hemispheres ○
c. hypothalamus ○
d. cerebellum. ○

2. Which of the following is NOT part of the meningeal membranes surrounding the brain?

a. dura mater ○
b. cisterna magna ○
c. pia mater ○
d. arachnoid mater. ○

3. Which cranial nerves supply the extrinsic muscles of the eye?

a. X, XII, I ○
b. V, VI, VII ○
c. III, IV, VI ○
d. I, II, III. ○

4. A sensory nerve may be defined as one that:

a. carries nerve impulses towards the CNS ○
b. lies between two nerves within the CNS ○
c. carries nerve impulses away from the CNS ○
d. supplies organs within the visceral body systems. ○

5. Which of the following is NOT a function of the sympathetic nervous system?

a. dilating the blood capillaries within the skeletal muscles ○
b. increasing secretion of saliva from the salivary glands ○
c. increasing the heart rate ○
d. increasing the rate of respiration. ○

6. In the eye, which of the following is NOT part of the uvea?

a. choroid ○
b. tapetum lucidum ○
c. iris ○
d. lens. ○

THE ANSWERS ARE:

1 d, 2 b, 3 c, 4 a, 5 b, 6 d.

5

The Endocrine System

The endocrine system is the second system of the body involved in the regulation of its functions, the first being the nervous system. In contrast to the nervous system, the response of which is rapid and lasts for a short period of time, the response of the endocrine system is much slower and in some cases may last for a lifetime. However, the two systems are equally important in maintaining homeostasis and work together to maintain a constant internal environment in a constantly changing external environment.

Memory Jogger

Homeostasis is the way in which the internal environment of the body is kept in a state of equilibrium so that all the body processes can work effectively. It involves osmoregulation, thermoregulation, respiration, buffers within the blood and excretion. Maintenance of homeostasis depends on information being sent to the brain from the nervous and endocrine systems.

The endocrine system consists of a series of **ductless or endocrine glands** whose secretions are known as **hormones**. These hormones are carried to their **target organ** by the bloodstream, so the target organ may be quite close by or some distance away. Hormones affect their chosen target organ – and no other – by being specifically structured to fit onto receptor sites on the target cell membranes.

Secretion of hormones is initiated by a specific stimulus, such as low levels of a blood constituent, e.g. calcium or by a nerve impulse, or by specific releasing hormones. Hormonal secretion is often controlled or 'switched off' by the presence of the hormone within the blood – this process is referred to as a **negative feedback loop**.

The endocrine glands are distributed around the body and their sites are shown in Fig. 5.1. The glands are:
- **Pituitary – the anterior and posterior** pituitary can be considered to be entirely separate glands. The pituitary is often described as the 'master gland' because it affects

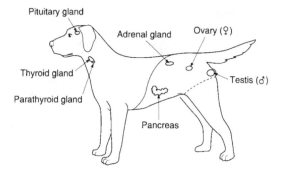

Figure 5.1 Components of the endocrine system

the actions of many other glands and forms a link with the nervous system.

- **Thyroid** – a pair of glands that secrete hormones affecting the metabolic rate of all the cells in the body and having an influence on blood calcium levels.
- **Parathyroid** – secretes a hormone that affects blood calcium levels.
- **Pancreas** – secretes three hormones that work together to regulate blood glucose.
- **Adrenal** – the **adrenal cortex and medulla** can be considered to be entirely separate glands. The cortex secretes about 30 different hormones, known as **corticosteroids**, which are divided into three groups according to their actions. The medulla secretes hormones that prepare the body for dangerous or stressful situations.
- **Ovary** – the female gonad. Secretes female reproductive hormones in a cycle known as the oestrous cycle. These affect the development of secondary sexual characteristics, behaviour, the production of ova, and pregnancy (see Chapter 10).
- **Testis** – the male gonad. Secretes male reproductive hormones, which affect the development of secondary sexual characteristics, behaviour and the production of spermatozoa (see Chapter 10).

The sites of the glands, actions of their hormones and the control of secretion are summarised in Table 5.1.

Table 5.1 The endocrine glands and their associated hormones

Endocrine gland	Location	Hormone	Function	Control of secretion
Anterior pituitary	Ventral to the forebrain	1. Thyroid stimulating hormone (TSH)	Stimulates the release of thyroid hormone	Hypothalamus
		2. Growth hormone or somatotrophin	Controls epiphyseal growth; protein production; regulates the use of energy	Hypothalamus
		3. Adrenocorticotrophic hormone (ACTH)	Controls the release of adrenocortical hormones	Hypothalamus
		4. Prolactin	Stimulates the development of mammary glands and secretion of milk	–
		5. Follicle stimulating hormone (FSH)	Stimulates the development of the ovarian follicles	Gonadotrophin releasing hormone from the hypothalamus (GRH)
		6. Luteinising hormone (LH)	Brings about ovulation of the ovarian follicles and development of the corpus luteum	Oestrogen secreted by Graafian follicles
		7. Interstitial cell stimulating hormone (ICSH)	Stimulates secretion of testosterone from the interstitial cells in the testis	Gonadotrophin releasing hormone from the hypothalamus (GRH)
Posterior pituitary	Ventral to the forebrain	1. Antidiuretic hormone (ADH) – vasopressin	Acts on the collecting ducts of the renal nephrons – changes the permeability to water	Status of the ECF and blood plasma

Table 5.1 (continued) The endocrine glands and their associated hormones

Endocrine gland	Location	Hormone	Function	Control of secretion
		2. Oxytocin	Stimulates uterine contractions during parturition and milk 'let down'	Suckling by the neonate initiates a reflex arc
Thyroid	Midline on the ventral aspect of the first few rings of the trachea	1. Thyroxin	Controls metabolic rate. Essential for normal growth	TSH
		2. Calcitonin	Decreases the resorption of calcium from bones	Raised blood calcium levels
Parathyroid	On either side of the thyroid gland	Parathormone	Stimulates calcium resorption from bones. Promotes calcium uptake from the intestine	Low blood calcium levels
Pancreas	Within the loop of the duodenum in the peritoneal cavity	1. Insulin – from the β cells in the islets of Langerhans	Increases uptake of glucose into the cells. Stores excess glucose as glycogen in the liver – glycogenesis	Raised blood glucose levels
		2. Glucagon – from the α cells in the islets of Langerhans	Breaks down glycogen stored in the liver to release glucose into the blood – glycogenolysis	Low blood glucose levels

Table 5.1 (continued) The endocrine glands and their associated hormones

Endocrine gland	Location	Hormone	Function	Control of secretion
		3. Somatostatin – from the δ cells in the Islets of Langerhans	Mild inhibition of insulin and glucagon, preventing swings in blood glucose levels. Decreases gut motility and secretion of digestive juices	–
Adrenal cortex	Cranial to the kidney in the peritoneal cavity – outer layer.	1. Glucocorticoids	Raise blood glucose levels. Reduce the inflammatory response.	ACTH
		2. Mineralocorticoids, e.g. aldosterone	Act on the distal convoluted tubules of the renal nephrons – regulate uptake of sodium and acid–base balance	Status of the ECF and blood plasma
		3. Sex hormones	Very small quantities	
Adrenal medulla	Cranial to the kidney in the peritoneal cavity – inner layer	Adrenaline and noradrenaline	Fear, flight, fright syndrome	Sympathetic nervous system

Table 5.1 (continued) The endocrine glands and their associated hormones

Endocrine gland	Location	Hormone	Function	Control of secretion
Ovary	One on either side of the midline in the dorsal peritoneal cavity	1. Oestrogen – from the Graafian follicles	Signs of oestrus; preparation of the reproductive tract and external genitalia for coitus.	FSH
		2. Progesterone – from the corpus luteum	Preparation of the reproductive tract for pregnancy; development of the mammary glands; maintains the pregnancy	LH
Testis	Outside the body cavity within the scrotum	Testosterone from the cells of Leydig	Spermatogenesis. Male secondary sexual characteristics and behaviour	ICSH

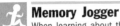

Memory Jogger

When learning about the endocrine glands and their hormones, consider the following:

· Site of the gland.
· What hormone(s) does it secrete?
· What stimulates secretion?
· What is the target organ?
· What effect does it have?
· What switches it off?

Table 5.1 will help you, but you will only revise successfully by making your own table.

There are many naturally occurring substances within the body that also have endocrine activity. These are not secreted by the major glands but are produced from tissues within other organs, such as the kidneys and the gastrointestinal tract. The most important hormones are:

- **Erythropoietin** – secreted by the kidneys in response to low levels of oxygen in the blood. It acts on the bone marrow and stimulates the production of new red blood cells.

- **Renin** – secreted by the glomeruli of the kidneys in response to low arterial blood pressure. It converts the plasma protein angiotensinogen into angiotensin, which initiates a series of reactions to raise the blood pressure (see Chapter 9).

- **Gastrin** – secreted by the walls of the stomach in response to muscle stretching as food passes through the cardiac sphincter. It stimulates the secretion of gastric juices from the gastric glands in the walls of the stomach (see Chapter 8).

- **Secretin** – secreted by the walls of the small intestine in response to muscle stretching as food passes through the pyloric sphincter into the duodenum. It stimulates the secretion of digestive enzymes from the exocrine part of the pancreas (see Chapter 8).

- **Cholecystokinin** – secreted by the walls of the duodenum and jejunum in response to the presence of food in the lumen of the small intestine. It causes the gall bladder to contract and release bile and also stimulates the secretion of digestive enzymes from the pancreas (see Chapter 8).

MULTIPLE CHOICE

Now use these multiple choice questions to test your understanding of this chapter.

1. Which of the following hormones is NOT produced by the anterior pituitary gland?

a. prolactin ○

b. FSH ○

c. oxytocin ○

d. TSH. ○

2. Which of the following statements about the endocrine glands is FALSE?

a. They secrete hormones that are specifically designed to affect one target organ and no other. ○

b. They may be controlled by the presence of hormones or other chemicals in the blood. ○

c. They secrete hormones directly into the bloodstream. ○

d. They secrete hormones into their target organ by means of a duct. ○

3. Which of the following are not classed as major endocrine glands?

a. kidney ○

b. adrenal ○

c. pituitary ○

d. pancreas. ○

4. The pancreas lies:

a. within the tissue of the brain ○

b. within the loop of the duodenum ○

c. close to the larynx in the neck ○

d. on the ventral surface of the forebrain. ○

5. Which of the following hormones has an effect on levels of glucose in the blood?

a. insulin ○

b. glucocorticoids ○

c. somatostatin ○

d. all of the above. ○

6. If blood calcium levels fall which hormone is released?

a. thyroxin   ○
b. parathormone   ○
c. vitamin D   ○
d. calcitonin.   ○

THE ANSWERS ARE:

1 c, 2 d, 3 a, 4 b, 5 d, 6 d.

6

The Blood-Vascular System

The blood-vascular system is distributed throughout the body. Its principal function is to deliver to all the cells and tissues of the body the nutrients needed for effective metabolism and for survival, and to collect the resulting waste materials. The system consists of four main parts, each of which contributes to the general function. If any of the individual components fails then the animal becomes ill or may even die.

The parts of the blood-vascular system are:
- **Blood** – a variety of cells within a liquid matrix. Each of the component parts is adapted to carry different materials or perform one of the other functions of blood.
- **Heart** – a muscular organ, which pumps blood around the body.
- **Circulatory system** – a series of linked vessels in which blood flows to all parts of the body and returns to the heart and lungs.
- **Lymphatic system** – a system of vessels that collect excess tissue fluid or lymph from the peripheral tissues and return it to the circulation.

THE BLOOD

The functions of blood can be divided into two major groups:
1. **Transport** – blood carries the following dissolved substances around the body:
- **Oxygen** diffuses from the inspired air within the lungs and is carried by haemoglobin in the erythrocytes to the tissues.
- **Carbon dioxide** produced by the tissues diffuses into the plasma and is carried in solution to the lungs, from which it is expired.
- **Nutrients** made available by digestion are carried to the liver for metabolism.

- **Waste products** produced by the tissues are carried to the liver and kidneys to be excreted.
- **Hormones** are carried from the endocrine glands to their target organs.

2. **Regulation** – blood is responsible for maintaining the internal equilibrium of the body – **homeostasis**. It:
- plays a role in **temperature control** by conducting heat from the core to the body surface
- maintains **water balance** by monitoring the volume and osmotic concentration of the body fluids and adjusting them in the kidney and by thirst
- maintains the **acid–base balance** at the optimum pH so that the body systems can function effectively
- contains **plasma proteins** – principally albumin, fibrinogen, prothrombin and globulins, molecules which are too large to pass through the capillary walls and so retain water within the circulation by osmosis; they are responsible for maintaining blood volume and blood pressure
- plays a part in the body's **defence system**, through the different types of leucocyte
- brings about **blood clotting** to prevent excessive loss of blood after injury.

Memory Jogger
Homeostasis is the way in which the internal environment of the body is kept in a state of equilibrium so that all the body processes can work effectively. It involves osmoregulation, thermoregulation, respiration, buffers within the blood and excretion. Maintenance of homeostasis depends on information being sent to the brain from the nervous and endocrine systems.

- Blood is a red fluid that is a brighter red colour when carrying oxygen (oxygenated) and darker when it has given up its oxygen to the tissues (deoxygenated).
- The normal pH of blood is 7.35–7.45.
- Blood accounts for about 7% of total body weight.

Blood is a liquid connective tissue that consists of:
- **Plasma** – a liquid matrix that makes up 55–70% of the blood and is part of the extracellular fluid (ECF) compartment (see Chapter 2). Plasma consists of 90% water, in which are dissolved most of the substances transported by

the blood to the cells, such as nutrients, hormones and carbon dioxide.

Plasma is extracted when blood is spun in a centrifuge. **Serum** is a yellow fluid that results when blood is allowed to clot naturally.

- **Cells and cellular fragments** – there are three main types of blood cell:

1. *Erythrocytes* – also called red blood corpuscles. Biconcave discs about 7 µm in diameter, with no nucleus and filled with haemoglobin, a red pigment that contains iron. The function of erythrocytes is to carry oxygen from the lungs to the tissues.

Erythrocytes are formed before birth by the liver, spleen and bone marrow and after birth by the bone marrow. They are released into the circulation and survive for approximately 120 days. At the end of their life they are removed and broken down by the spleen or the lymph nodes. The formation of erythrocytes is regulated by the hormone erythropoietin, secreted by the kidneys in response to low oxygen levels in the blood (see Chapter 5).

- **erythropoiesis** – formation of erythrocytes
- **haemopoiesis** – formation of all parts of the blood
- **anaemia** – reduction in the number of erythrocytes.

2. *Leucocytes* – also called white blood cells. These are larger than erythrocytes and can be divided into two groups by examination of their cytoplasm:

   (a) **Granulocytes** – all have granules within the cytoplasm. Also called polymorphonucleocytes or PMNs. They make up 70% of all leucocytes. There are three types:

      - **Neutrophils** – form 90% of all granulocytes. Their nucleus is multilobed; granules take up neutral dyes and stain purple. Immature cells or **band cells** have a curved nucleus. Able to move into the tissues through the capillary walls to engulf invading bacteria or remove debris by phagocytosis. **Neutrophilia** means increased numbers of neutrophils, seen in bacterial infections. **Neutropenia** means decreased numbers of neutrophils, seen in some viral infections.

• **Eosinophils** – the nucleus is multilobed; granules take up acid dyes and stain red. They secrete enzymes that inactivate histamine and are involved in fighting and controlling parasitic and allergic reactions. **Eosinophilia** means increased number of eosinophils in response to parasitic infections.

• **Basophils** – present in very small numbers in the blood. The nucleus is multilobed; granules take up alkaline dyes and stain dark blue. They secrete histamine, which increases the inflammatory response, and heparin, which prevents unnecessary blood clotting.

(b) **Agranulocytes** – contain clear cytoplasm. There are two types:

• **Lymphocytes** – make up 80% of all agranulocytes. The nucleus is round and almost fills the cell. They originate from stem cells in the bone marrow and are differentiated in lymphoid tissue. They secrete antibodies and are responsible for the specific immune response.
• **Monocytes** – largest of the leucocytes but present in small numbers. They have a large horseshoe-shaped nucleus. They are phagocytic cells that are able to migrate to the tissues, where they are known as macrophages.

3. *Thrombocytes* – also called **platelets**. These are cell pieces formed by the fragmentation in the bone marrow of large cells called **megakaryocytes**. They play an essential part in the clotting process. **Thrombocytopenia** means lack of platelets.

BLOOD CLOTTING

This is an important part of the body's ability to limit injury and prevent blood loss and results in the formation of a clot that seals the damaged area.

The formation of a clot involves a series of complicated inter-linked chemical reactions and requires the presence of the plasma proteins prothrombin and fibrinogen, and calcium and vitamin K. Platelets stick to the damaged area and a network of fibrin develops; these trap the blood cells and a clot is formed.

Clotting time in a normal healthy animal is about 3–5 minutes but may be increased by factors such as movement of the wound edges, genetic factors such as haemophilia, low blood calcium, thrombocytopenia and lack of vitamin K.

 Memory Jogger
To simplify learning the functions of each of the blood cells, reduce them to a few words:
Erythrocytes or red blood cells – carry oxygen.
Neutrophils – remove bacteria and other debris by phagocytosis.
Eosinophils – control parasitic infections and allergic reactions.
Basophils – secrete histamine and heparin to prevent clotting.
Lymphocytes – secrete antibodies as part of the specific immune response.
Monocytes – remove debris by phagocytosis.
Thrombocytes – blood clotting.

THE HEART

The heart is a muscular organ, which pumps blood around the body within the circulatory system (Fig. 6.1). It lies within the mediastinum of the thoracic cavity, occupying a more or less central position but with the apex angled slightly to the left. Externally on the chest wall, it extends from approximately the third rib to the caudal border of the sixth rib.

The heart consists of four chambers. These are the:
- right and left **atria** (singular, atrium)
- right and left **ventricles**.

The right side of the heart is separated from the left by a wall or **interventricular septum**.

STRUCTURE OF THE HEART WALL

From the inside out there are three layers:

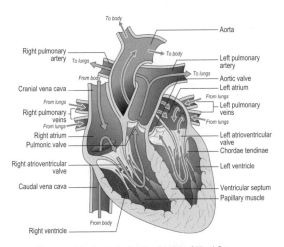

Figure 6.1 Structure of the heart showing the direction of blood flow

1. A single layer of epithelial cells forming a lining known as the **endocardium**. This is continuous with the lining of all the blood vessels, which is called the **endothelium**.
2. A thick layer of cardiac muscle known as the **myocardium**, which is capable of rhythmic contraction throughout life (see Chapter 2).
3. An outer double layer of epithelial cells known as the **pericardium**. Between these two layers of cells is the **pericardial cavity or sac**. This contains a small volume of serous lubricating fluid secreted by the epithelial cells.

HEART VALVES

In order to ensure that blood follows the correct route through the heart, there are two sets of valves within the chambers of the heart. These are the:

1. **Atrioventricular valves (AV valves)** – these lie between the atria and ventricles on either side of the heart (Fig. 6.1):
- **right AV valve** – has three flaps or **cusps** and is also known as the **tricuspid valve**

- **left AV valve** – has two cusps and is also known as the **bicuspid or mitral valve**.

The free edges of the cusps are attached to the myocardium by fibrous threads known as **chordae tendinae**. These prevent the valves being turned inside out by the force of the blood flow during heart contraction.

2. **Semilunar valves** (so called because they are half-moon shaped) – these lie at the base of the major arteries carrying blood away from the heart (Fig. 6.1):
- **pulmonic valve** – at the base of the pulmonary artery, leading from the right ventricle to the lungs
- **aortic valve** – at the base of the aorta, leading from the left ventricle to the systemic circulation.

DIRECTION OF BLOOD FLOW THROUGH THE HEART

To make this easier to understand, we will follow the blood flow through one side of the heart at a time. In reality, both sides of the heart are contracting and relaxing at the same time. The following sequence of events, known as the **cardiac cycle**, makes up a complete heartbeat.

- Blood enters the **right atrium** of the heart from the systemic circulation via **the cranial and caudal venae cavae**.
- The right atrium contracts and blood is forced into the **right ventricle** through the open **right AV valve**.
- The right ventricle contracts and blood is forced against the underside of the AV valve. This closes the valve, preventing blood from flowing back into the atrium. Blood flows out of the ventricle into the **pulmonary artery** and then to the lungs in the **pulmonary circulation**, where it becomes oxygenated.
- As the right ventricle relaxes the **pulmonic valve** closes, preventing blood from flowing back into the ventricle.
- Oxygenated blood returns from the lungs and enters the **left atrium** via the **pulmonary veins**.
- The left atrium contracts and blood is forced into the **left ventricle** through the open **left AV valve**.
- The left ventricle contracts and blood is forced against the underside of the AV valve. This closes the valve, preventing blood from flowing back into the atrium. Blood flows

out of the ventricle into the **aorta** and then around the body in the **systemic circulation**.

- As the left ventricle relaxes the **aortic valve** closes, preventing blood from flowing back into the ventricle.

The contractile phase of the atria and ventricles is known as **systole** (pronounced sis-stol-i).

The relaxation phase of the atria and ventricles is known as **diastole** (pronounced dias-stol-i).

Memory Jogger
To relate the physiology of the heart to the sound you can hear through a stethoscope - a process called **auscultation**:
The first heart sound - 'lub' - is due to the closure of the atrioventricular valves.
The second heart sound - 'dub' - is due to the closure of the semilunar valves.

Memory Jogger
The physiological state of an animal can be assessed by measuring the number of times that the heart beats per minute. This is the **pulse rate or heart rate**. The normal value for a dog is 70–120 per minute and for a cat it is 120–180 per minute.

NERVOUS CONTROL OF THE CARDIAC CYCLE

Cardiac muscle has the intrinsic ability to contract rhythmically without nervous input, but in order to satisfy the changing needs of the body, the heart must be able to alter rapidly the rate at which it beats. This is brought about by the autonomic nervous system - the vagus nerve (cranial nerve X), which contains parasympathetic nerve fibres, slows the heart rate and sympathetic nerve fibres increase the rate.

Within the tissue of the heart there is a **conduction system** of nervous tissue which is responsible for initiating and coordinating the heartbeat. This consists of:

- the **sinoatrial node** within the wall of the right atrium
- the **atrioventricular node** at the top of the interventricular septum
- the **bundle of His** within the tissue of the interventricular septum
- **Purkinje fibres**, forming a network of specialised cells within the walls of the ventricles.

Nerve impulses from the autonomic nervous system stimulate the sinoatrial node, which is often known as the pacemaker of the heart. The nerve impulses spread across the walls of the right atrium, stimulate the atrioventricular node and pass down the bundle of His. They then stimulate the Purkinje fibres, causing a wave of muscle contraction to begin in the ventricular myocardium at the apex of the heart; this forces blood upwards and out via the pulmonary arteries and the aorta.

THE CIRCULATORY SYSTEM

Blood flows around the body and back to the heart in a series of linked blood vessels. Most blood vessels have a similar structure, consisting of three layers of tissue, but these vary in size and thickness (Table 6.1). Working from the inside out they are:

- **Tunica intima** – a single layer of epithelial cells known as the **endothelium**. This is continuous throughout the entire circulatory system, including the inner layer of the heart, where it is known as the **endocardium**.
- **Tunica media** – consists of smooth muscle and elastic tissue.
- **Tunica adventitia** – the fibrous outer covering.

The route of the blood vessels is continuous, so that the **arteries** carry blood away from the heart and branch off to form smaller **arterioles**, which lead into **capillaries** within the tissues. Eventually the capillaries join up to form **venules**; these combine to form the larger **veins**, which drain blood *back* into the heart. If a blockage develops at any point in this network, side or **collateral vessels** develop to form an **anastomosis**, which bypasses the blockage and ensures the affected tissue receives its vital blood supply.

 Memory Jogger
ARTERIES carry blood AWAY from the heart.
VEINS carry blood TOWARDS the heart.

The circulatory system can be divided into two subsystems:

1. **Pulmonary circulation** – the **pulmonary artery** carries deoxygenated blood from the heart to the lungs, where it becomes oxygenated. It is then returned to the heart in the **pulmonary veins**.

Table 6.1 Structure of blood vessels

Blood vessels	Structure	Function
Arteries	Large vessels with thick walls that enable the arteries to withstand the pressure of blood leaving the heart. Able to constrict and dilate in response to the needs of the body	Carry oxygenated blood away from the heart. *The exception is the pulmonary artery, which carries deoxygenated blood*
Arterioles	Within the deeper tissues the arteries divide to form these smaller and thinner-walled vessels	Carry oxygenated blood and nutrients to the tissues
Capillaries	Arterioles divide to form these very narrow, thin-walled vessels deep within the tissues. Walls consist of a single layer of endothelial cells. Arrangement of capillaries is called the capillary bed or capillary network	Deliver all nutrients and oxygen to the cells and collect waste products. Thin walls allow materials to diffuse in and out of the blood
Venules	Capillaries combine to form these thicker-walled vessels as they leave the deeper tissues	Carry deoxygenated blood and waste products produced by the tissues
Veins	Large vessels that have a thinner wall and a larger lumen than an artery. Some veins, e.g. those in the legs, have valves to prevent backflow of blood against gravity	Carry deoxygenated blood to the heart. *The exception is the pulmonary vein, which carries oxygenated blood*

2. **Systemic circulation** – the arterial circulation takes oxygenated blood from the heart around the body to the tissues and the venous circulation returns de-oxygenated blood to the heart.

Arterial circulation – the major artery of the body is the **aorta**. As it leaves the left ventricle of the heart it gives off arteries in the following order:
- A pair of **coronary arteries** supply the heart muscle.
- The **brachiocephalic trunk** supplies the head and neck via a pair of **common carotids** and the **right subclavian artery** supplies the right forelimb.

- The **left subclavian artery** supplies the left forelimb.
- Paired **spinal arteries** supply the region of the thoracic vertebrae and muscles.
- A pair of **renal arteries** supply the kidneys.
- A pair of **ovarian or testicular (spermatic) arteries** supply the female or male gonads.
- Three large unpaired arteries – the **coeliac, cranial mesenteric** and **caudal mesenteric** – supply the stomach and intestinal tract.
- A pair of **external iliac arteries** supply the hind limb.
- A pair of **internal iliac arteries** supply the pelvic viscera.

Venous circulation – the veins drain blood into the right ventricle of the heart via two major veins – the cranial vena cava and caudal vena cava – and a smaller vessel, the azygous vein:

- **Cranial vena cava** – collects blood from the head and neck via a pair of **jugular veins** and from the forelimbs via the right and left **subclavian veins.**
- **Caudal vena cava** – collects blood from the pelvic viscera, hind limbs and abdominal organs via veins that follow a broadly similar pattern to the arteries.
- **Azygous vein** – a smaller vein that collects blood from the thoracic body wall and either joins the cranial vena cava or enters directly into the right atrium.

Memory Jogger

Most arteries and veins are paired and are named after the organ they supply, which makes it much easier to remember them.

Hepatic portal system – this is part of the systemic circulation but is an adaptation that enables the products of digestion to be transported via the **hepatic portal vein** from the small intestine straight to the liver to be metabolised. Oxygenated blood reaches the liver via the hepatic artery and deoxygenated blood leaves the liver in the **hepatic vein** (see Chapter 8).

THE LYMPHATIC SYSTEM

The **functions** of the lymphatic system are to:

1. drain lymph from the interstitial spaces in the tissues and return it to the circulation

2. filter foreign bodies (e.g. bacteria) from the lymph
3. produce lymphocytes and antibodies as part of the body's specific immune response
4. transport digested fat by means of the lacteals in the intestinal wall.

Lymph – excess tissue fluid that leaks out of the capillaries to fill the interstitial spaces and bathe the cells. Some passes back into the capillaries but the remainder is collected by the lymphatic drainage. It is similar in composition to plasma but contains less protein and more lymphocytes.

The **parts** of the lymphatic system are:

- **Lymphatic capillaries** – thin-walled channels creating a network throughout the tissues. The **lacteals**, which lie within the villi of the small intestinal wall, are a type of lymphatic capillary (see Chapter 8). Lymph drains from the tissues into the capillaries, which combine to form the lymphatic vessels.
- **Lymphatic vessels** – similar in structure to the veins. Some vessels also have valves to maintain a one-way flow away from the tissues. Contraction of the surrounding muscles helps to propel the fluid towards the heart.

  Major lymphatic vessels are:
  - **Thoracic duct** – starts in the dorsal anterior abdomen as the **cisterna chyli**, runs cranially through the thorax and drains into one of the major veins opening into the right atrium; drains lymph from the hind limbs, lumbar region, lacteals and the left forelimb and chest.
  - **Right lymphatic duct** – drains lymph from the right forelimb and the right side of the chest and opens into the cranial vena cava or the right jugular vein.
  - **Tracheal ducts** – a pair of ducts that drain the head and neck and open into the same sites as the other vessels.

Lymph nodes – as lymph is carried along the lymph vessels it passes through lymph nodes, whose function is to filter and monitor any foreign material that has been picked up in the lymph. Within the node, lymphocytes form specific antibodies to the foreign material and the node becomes enlarged as a result of this 'challenge'.

Each node consists of an encapsulated mass of lymphoid tissue supported by connective tissue **trabeculae**. On the outside many **afferent vessels** carry lymph into the node and the lymph leaves by one **efferent vessel**.

Each region of the body and each organ has its own lymph node. Some are deep in the tissues but some are more superficial and can be palpated to assess the degree of local infection. The palpable lymph nodes are:

- **submandibular** – at the edge of the angle of the jaw
- **parotid** – just caudal to the temporo-mandibular joint of the jaw
- **superficial cervical or prescapular nodes** – just in front of the shoulder joint at the base of the neck
- **superficial inguinal** – in the groin between the thigh and the abdominal body wall
- **popliteal** – within the tissue of the gastrocnemius muscle (see Chapter 3), caudal to the stifle joint.

Memory Jogger

It is important to remember the sites of the palpable lymph nodes as they are a useful diagnostic tool. The best way to learn them is to use a live animal and relate the theory to real life – start palpating them!

Lymph follicles – small masses of lymphoid tissue distributed within other organs, e.g. the intestinal tract.

Larger lymphoid structures

- **Tonsils** – form a ring around the junction of the oral cavity and pharynx. The largest one is the palatine tonsil.
- **Thymus gland** – lies in the thoracic inlet and the cranial part of the thoracic cavity. Atrophies and is replaced by fat during the first year of life. It is the site of the differentiation of the T lymphocytes involved in cell-mediated immunity.
- **Spleen** – a large, deep red haemopoietic organ closely attached to the greater curvature of the stomach. It stores erythrocytes, removes old erythrocytes, produces lymphocytes and removes foreign material from the circulation. However, it is not essential for life and may have to be removed if affected by disease or trauma.

MULTIPLE CHOICE

Now use these multiple choice questions to test your understanding of this chapter.

1. The granulocytes in the blood consist of which of the following cells?

a. eosinophils, platelets and monocytes ○

b. basophils, neutrophils and eosinophils ○

c. monocytes, lymphocytes and platelets ○

d. erythrocytes, lymphocytes and neutrophils. ○

2. The route taken by the blood as it flows through the heart is:

a. left atrium, left ventricle, pulmonary artery, pulmonary vein, right atrium, right ventricle, aorta ○

b. right ventricle, pulmonary vein, left atrium, left ventricle, aorta ○

c. right atrium, right ventricle, pulmonary artery, pulmonary vein, left atrium, left ventricle, aorta ○

d. aorta, right ventricle, right atrium, pulmonary vein, pulmonary artery, right ventricle, right atrium. ○

3. The mitral valve of the heart is also known as the:

a. tricuspid valve ○

b. pulmonic valve ○

c. aortic valve ○

d. left atrioventricular valve. ○

4. Which part of the conduction system of the heart is in direct contact with nerves of the autonomic nervous system?

a. sinoatrial node ○

b. bundle of His ○

c. atrioventricular node ○

d. Purkinje fibres. ○

5. Blood is collected from the thoracic body wall by which vein?

a. jugular ○
b. cranial vena cava ○
c. azygous vein ○
d. spinal vein. ○

6. Which lymph node is located within the gastro-cnemius muscle?

a. parotid ○
b. superficial inguinal ○
c. prescapular ○
d. popliteal. ○

THE ANSWERS ARE:

1 b, 2 c, 3 d, 4 a, 5 c, 6 d.

7

The Respiratory System

The respiratory system lies within the head, neck and thorax. It is relatively straightforward and one of the easiest systems to understand, because, as you learn about the parts and what they do, you can feel yourself breathing and controlling your respiratory rate. Nervous control of the system is more complicated and requires a bit more thought!

First let's sort out the **components** of respiration.

- **Respiration** – the exchange of gases between a living organism and its environment. This can be divided into two stages:

  - **External respiration** – the exchange of gases between the inspired atmospheric air within the lungs and the blood of the organism. This is also called **breathing**.

  - **Internal respiration** – the exchange of gases between the blood and the tissues. This is also called **tissue respiration**.

The **functions** of the respiratory system are to:

- conduct inspired air containing oxygen from the external atmosphere to the site of gaseous exchange within the lungs

- conduct air containing carbon dioxide produced by the tissues from the site of gaseous exchange to the external atmosphere.

THE RESPIRATORY TRACT

The parts of the respiratory tract are:

- nose and nasal chambers
- pharynx
- larynx
- trachea
- bronchi and bronchioles
- alveolar ducts and alveoli.

The **upper respiratory tract** comprises the nasal chambers, pharynx, larynx and the part of the trachea within the neck. The **lower respiratory tract** comprises the trachea as it runs through the thorax and the lungs.

- **Nose and nasal chambers** – the nasal cavity is formed by the maxilla, incisive, nasal and palatine bones of the skull (see Chapter 3). It is divided into the right and left **nasal chambers** by a cartilaginous **nasal septum**. Inspired air enters the chambers via the **external nares** or nostrils and leaves via the **internal nares**, where it enters the pharynx. The external nares are protected by a pad of stratified pigmented squamous epithelium known as the **rhinarium**.

The two nasal chambers are partially filled with coiled **ethmoturbinates or conchae**. These delicate bones are covered in **ciliated mucous membrane**, which has a good blood supply and serves to moisten and warm the inspired air. The cilia filter the air and trap any particles in the covering of mucus, preventing them from reaching the lower respiratory tract. The epithelium covering the dorsocaudal part of the nasal chambers forms the **olfactory mucosa**, which is responsible for olfaction (see Chapter 4).

Leading from each nasal chamber is a pair of **sinuses** – the **frontal sinus** within the frontal bone of the skull and the **maxillary sinus** within the maxillary and palatine bones. These are air-filled cavities lined with mucous membrane whose function is to warm, moisten and filter the inspired air and to reduce the weight of the skull.

- **Pharynx** – a muscular tube lined with mucous membrane which forms a crossover point between the respiratory and digestive systems. The soft palate extends caudally and divides the pharynx into the **nasopharynx** at the back of the nasal chambers and the **oropharynx** at the back of the oral cavity. Leading from the pharynx are the **larynx** and **trachea** and the **oesophagus**. Opening into the wall of the pharynx are the **eustachian tubes**, one leading from each middle ear. Within the walls of the pharynx are deposits of lymphoid tissue known as the **tonsils** (see Chapter 8).
- **Larynx** – a complex collection of three single cartilages,

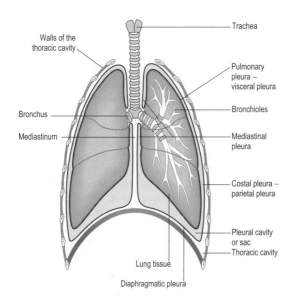

Walls of the
thoracic cavity

Trachea

Pulmonary
pleura –
visceral pleura

Bronchus

Bronchioles

Mediastinum

Mediastinal
pleura

Costal pleura –
parietal pleura

Pleural cavity
or sac

Thoracic cavity

Lung tissue

Diaphragmatic pleura

Figure 7.1 Longitudinal section through the thoracic cavity

one pair of interconnected cartilages, muscle and connective tissue forming a rigid hollow structure that controls the flow of gases into the respiratory tract and prevents the entry of any solid matter. It is also involved in vocalisation. The larynx lies in the midline and is attached to the skull by the **hyoid apparatus**, which enables it to swing backwards and forwards during breathing and swallowing.

- The most rostral cartilage, the **epiglottis**, is attached to the ventral border of the larynx and closes the opening of the larynx or the **glottis** during swallowing. Inside the larynx is a pair of **vocal folds**, the outer edges of which are the **vocal cords**. These are able to move, and either lie flat against the wall of the larynx or partially obstruct the lumen so that air passing over the vocal cords creates sound.
- **Trachea** – a permanently open tube that conducts air from the larynx into the bronchi (Fig. 7.1). It runs through the thoracic cavity and divides just above the heart into the

right and left bronchi. The tube consists of a series of C-shaped hyaline cartilages linked by smooth muscle and connective tissue, and it is lined with ciliated mucous membrane.

- **Bronchi** – the right and left bronchi are of a similar structure to the trachea except that the two tubes are of a smaller diameter and the cartilaginous rings are complete. Each bronchus enters the lung tissue at a point known as the root of the lung.

- **Bronchioles** – within the lungs the bronchi divide into bronchioles, which continue to divide, getting smaller and smaller (Fig. 7.1). The larger bronchioles are kept open by cartilage rings but in the smaller ones the cartilage disappears. The smallest bronchioles are known as **respiratory bronchioles**. All the tubes are lined with ciliated mucous membrane. This arrangement of bronchi and bronchioles is referred to as the **bronchial tree**.

- **Alveolar ducts and alveoli** – eventually each respiratory bronchiole gives rise to several **alveolar ducts**, which terminate in blind-ending sacs or alveoli. The alveolar ducts and alveoli are lined with the **pulmonary membrane**, which is a single cell thick and is not ciliated. Gaseous exchange takes place across this membrane. Each alveolus is covered with a network of thin-walled blood capillaries, which are part of the pulmonary circulation (see Chapter 6).

Gross appearance of the lungs – the lungs are two pale pink, spongy organs, which almost fill the thoracic cavity. There is no muscle within the lung tissue but it does contain elastic tissue, which allows it to return to its original shape after expanding with air. Each lung is divided by deep fissures into **lobes**, each of which is named according to its site. The right lung is larger than the left (Table 7.1).

THE THORACIC CAVITY

The thoracic cavity is a bony cage lined with a thin serous membrane known as the **pleura**, creating the **pleural cavity** (Fig. 7.1) (see Chapters 2 and 3). The pleural cavity is divided into the right and left pleural cavities by the **mediastinum**, which contains most of the thoracic organs and their associated blood vessels and nerves (Table 7.2).

Table 7.1 The lobes of the lung

Right lung	Left lung
Apical or cranial lobe	Apical or cranial lobe
Cardiac or middle lobe	Cardiac or middle lobe
Diaphragmatic or caudal lobe	Diaphragmatic lobe or caudal lobe
Accessory lobe	No accessory lobe

Table 7.2 Structures within the mediastinum

Transverse section through thoracic cavity	Organs in this part of the mediastinum
Cranial section	Oesophagus, trachea, cranial vena cava, aorta
Middle section	Oesophagus, trachea (or right and left bronchi), heart
Caudal section	Oesophagus, caudal vena cava, aorta

Table 7.3 The pleural membranes

Pleural membrane	Area covered
Pulmonary or visceral	Lungs
Parietal – subdivided into:	Inner surface of the thoracic cavity
• Mediastinal	Mediastinum
• Costal	Ribs
• Diaphragmatic	Diaphragm

The right and left lungs and the lower part of their principal bronchi lie within the right and left pleural cavities. The pleura covers all the structures within the pleural cavities and the parts of it are named according to the area it covers (Table 7.3).

The pleural cavity lies between the pulmonary pleura and the parietal pleura and contains nothing but a vacuum and a small amount of serous fluid. This fluid serves to lubricate the movements of the lungs and the thoracic wall.

THE MECHANICS OF RESPIRATION

There are three aspects that must be considered.

1. How does the animal take in and expel air, i.e. how does it breathe?
2. How is oxygen transferred from the lungs to the tissues and how is carbon dioxide collected from the tissues and transferred to the lungs, i.e. how does gaseous exchange occur?
3. How are these actions controlled and coordinated?

BREATHING

Breathing requires the actions of two sets of muscles (see Chapter 3):

- **External and internal intercostal muscles** – skeletal muscles running in two layers between the ribs and forming the lateral walls of the thorax. Innervated by the **intercostal nerves**.
- **Diaphragm** – the large dome-shaped muscle forming the caudal boundary of the thoracic cavity. Innervated by the **phrenic nerve**.

Air is able to enter the lungs only when the pressure of the external air is greater than the pressure within the lungs. The lungs are totally enclosed and surrounded by a vacuum within the pleural cavity.

Breathing takes place in two stages:

1. **Inspiration** – this is an active process.
   - The diaphragm contracts and flattens.
   - The external intercostal muscles contract and lift the ribs upwards and outwards.

   The net result is an **increase in the volume** of the thoracic cavity, which causes a **reduction in pressure** within the cavity. The lungs expand and air rushes down the trachea into the lungs.

2. **Expiration** – this is mainly a passive process.
   - The diaphragm relaxes and curves upwards.
   - The external intercostal muscles relax and the ribs drop down.

Table 7.4 Percentage of gases in inspired and expired air

Gas	Inspired air	Expired air
Nitrogen	79%	79%
Oxygen	21%	16%
Carbon dioxide	0.04%	4–5%
Water vapour	Depends on many factors	Increased because of insensible water loss
Other gases	Trace	Trace

The net result is a **decrease in the volume** of the thoracic cavity, which causes an **increase in pressure** within the cavity. The lungs collapse and air is pushed up the trachea and out of the body.

During **forced expiration** the internal intercostals and the abdominal muscles contract to push air out of the lungs with great force.

Memory Jogger
Now try this. As you read the description of breathing, place your hands over your ribs and breathe in. You will feel your ribs go upwards and outwards. Now breathe out and feel them drop down. Just remember that it is the movements of the rib cage and diaphragm that make the air go in and out, not the other way round, as you might have thought.

GASEOUS EXCHANGE
The composition of inspired and expired air is shown in Table 7.4.

The process of gaseous exchange takes place across the pulmonary membrane lining the alveoli:
1. Oxygen within the inspired air is conducted down the respiratory tract to the alveoli, each of which is surrounded by a network of blood capillaries.
2. Within the alveoli the concentration of oxygen is high but it is low in the blood capillaries, so oxygen diffuses from the alveoli into the blood.
3. The blood, now oxygenated, is pumped away in the pulmonary veins towards the heart and around the body in the systemic circulation.

4. Deoxygenated blood carrying carbon dioxide produced by the tissues is pumped by the heart to the lungs in the pulmonary arteries and then in the pulmonary capillaries, which surround the alveoli.

5. Within the capillaries the concentration of carbon dioxide is high but it is low in the alveoli, so carbon dioxide diffuses from the blood into the alveoli.

6. Carbon dioxide is then conducted up the respiratory tract and is breathed out in the expired air.

CONTROL OF RESPIRATION

This is done by the nervous system and is designed to ensure the supply of oxygen to the tissues in response to the changing demands of the body's metabolism.

- **Central control** is brought about by respiratory control centres within the pons and medulla oblongata of the hindbrain (see Chapter 4).
  - The **apneustic** and **pneumotaxic centres** control expiration.
  - The **inspiratory centre** controls inspiration.

The centres inhibit each other and cannot work simultaneously. They control the basic **rhythm** of respiration.

  - Nerve impulses from the inspiratory centre travel along the **phrenic nerve** to the diaphragm and the intercostal nerves to the **intercostal muscles**. The muscles contract and inspiration occurs.
  - Expiration is mainly passive but some nerve impulses from the apneustic and pneumotaxic centres may cause contraction of the internal intercostal muscles and assist in expiration.

- **Peripheral control** occurs by means of receptors distributed throughout the body. These control the **rate and depth** of respiration.
  - **Stretch receptors** lie within the walls of the bronchi and bronchioles. As air passes into the lungs, nerve impulses are transmitted from the receptors to the inspiratory centre in the medulla oblongata via the vagus nerve (X). This inhibits further inspiration and stimulates expiration, preventing overinflation of the lungs. This is known as the

Hering–Breuer reflex.

- **Chemoreceptors** – there are two types:

  - **peripheral** – **carotid bodies** within the wall of the carotid artery and **aortic bodies** within the wall of the aorta close to the heart

  - **central** – within the medulla oblongata of the hind brain.

Chemoreceptors monitor the concentration of oxygen and carbon dioxide in the blood. Low levels of oxygen stimulate the inspiratory centres so that more oxygen is taken in, while changes in carbon dioxide levels will alter the pH of the blood, which will either inhibit or stimulate inspiration. Monitoring pH is an essential part of homeostasis as most body processes will only function effectively within a pH range of 7.35–7.45.

Memory Jogger

Homeostasis is the way in which the internal environment of the body is kept in a state of equilibrium so that all the body processes can work effectively. It involves osmoregulation, thermoregulation, respiration, buffers within the blood, and excretion. Maintenance of homeostasis depends on information being sent to the brain from the nervous and endocrine systems.

The relationship between the inspiratory and expiratory centres in the brain and the peripheral receptors controls respiration and enables the respiratory system to respond to the changing metabolic demands of the body.

MULTIPLE CHOICE

Now use these multiple choice questions to test your understanding of this chapter.

1. The nasal cavity is filled with:

a. sinuses   ◯

b. ethmoturbinates   ◯

c. alveoli   ◯

d. nasal septum.   ◯

2. Compared with inhaled air, exhaled air contains:

a. less oxygen ○

b. less nitrogen ○

c. more oxygen ○

d. less carbon dioxide. ○

3. The Eustachian tube connects the pharynx with the:

a. nasal cavity ○

b. oesophagus ○

c. middle ear ○

d. frontal sinus. ○

4. Gaseous exchange occurs within the:

a. trachea ○

b. bronchi ○

c. respiratory bronchioles ○

d. alveoli. ○

5. Which nerve controls the movement of the diaphragm?

a. intercostal nerve ○

b. phrenic nerve ○

c. spinal nerve ○

d. vagus nerve. ○

6. The Hering–Breuer reflex is concerned with:

a. levels of carbon dioxide in the expired air ○

b. the degree of stretch in the walls of the bronchi and bronchioles ○

c. pH of the blood ○

d. the osmotic concentration of the body fluids. ○

THE ANSWERS ARE:

1 b, 2 a, 3 c, 4 d, 5 b, 6 b.

8

The Digestive System

All living organisms must have energy to fuel the activities performed by the body. The source of this energy is food. The digestive system has evolved to break down food materials into small units that can be absorbed into the blood and then processed to extract and make use of the energy. So, as you tuck into your burger and chips, you know what is happening to them!

The **functions** of the digestive system are to:
1. ingest, prehend or take food into the body
2. masticate or chew the food, enabling it to be swallowed
3. digest or break down the food into its basic chemical components
4. absorb the components into the bloodstream
5. metabolise the components to produce energy.

Within the class Mammalia there are several **types of digestive system**, which are adapted to deal with a range of foods.
1. **Carnivores** – flesh-eaters, such as dogs and cats. The teeth are sharp and pointed and adapted for tearing flesh from the bone. The intestinal tract is relatively short as meat is easily digested and takes little time. The stomach is single-chambered or **simple**, and digestion is described as **monogastric**.
2. **Herbivores** – plant-eaters. Teeth are flattened 'table teeth', designed to grind up the tough vegetation. The length of the intestinal tract is long because plant material takes a long time to digest. Part of the digestive system is adapted to form a **fermentation chamber**, in which the cellulose cell walls of plants are broken down by the enzyme cellulase, produced by colonies of microorganisms living in the gut. Herbivores are subdivided into two groups according to the site of this chamber:
   • **Cranial fermenters or ruminants**, e.g. cattle, sheep, goats and deer. The stomach is four-chambered or **compound**. One part of the stomach, the **rumen**, is enlarged to form a fermentation chamber.

- **Caudal or hindgut fermenters**, e.g. rabbits, guinea-pigs and horses (see Chapter 13). An enlarged **caecum**, part of the large intestine, is adapted to form a fermentation chamber. The stomach is simple.

3. **Omnivores**, such as the pig, humans, the rat and the gerbil, eat any type of food (see Chapter 13). The teeth are a mixture of sharp teeth for cutting and flattened teeth for grinding. The length of the intestinal tract is intermediate between that of carnivores and herbivores. There is no fermentation chamber.

The digestive system consists of several parts, each of which contributes to the overall process. The **parts of the system** are:
- oral cavity – including lips, tongue, teeth and palate
- pharynx
- oesophagus
- stomach
- small intestine – duodenum, jejunum, ileum
- large intestine – caecum, colon, rectum, anal canal
- accessory structures – salivary glands, liver, pancreas, gall bladder.

THE ORAL CAVITY

Also called the **mouth or buccal cavity**. This is the opening to the digestive tract and consists of the lips, tongue, salivary glands and teeth. Its **functions** are to:
1. Pick up food using the lips and tongue.
2. Break up food into bite-sized pieces ready for swallowing. Food is made into a bolus by the movements of the tongue, teeth and cheeks.
3. Lubricate each bolus with saliva from the salivary glands so that it is easier to swallow.
4. Regulate temperature – saliva evaporates from the tongue during panting and it is also applied to the coat during grooming. Both of these have a cooling effect.
5. Make sounds – involves the tongue and lips.
6. Taste food, using the taste buds on the tongue and pharynx.

The oral cavity is formed by the lower jaw or **right and left**

mandibles and the upper jaw or **maxilla and incisive bones**. The **palatine bone or hard palate** forms the roof of the mouth (and the floor of the nasal cavity) and is extended caudally as the **soft palate** (see Chapter 3).

The sides of the jaws are connected by skin that is lined on the inside with mucous membrane. Between these two layers are the **masseter muscle**, which forms the cheek and is responsible for closing the jaw (see Chapter 3). The entire cavity is lined with mucous membrane, which reflects onto the jaw bones as the **gums or periodontal membrane** and is pierced by the teeth, forming the sockets or alveoli.

- **Lips** – consist of muscle covered in skin and lined with mucous membrane. The upper lip is split vertically by a deep **philtrum** and bears the sensitive **whiskers or vibrissae**.
- **Tongue** – consists of a mass of striated muscle fibres running in all directions, some of which are attached to the hyoid apparatus and some to the mandible, forming the root, which is continuous with the larynx. The tip is unattached and very mobile. The tongue is covered with mucous membrane arranged in **papillae**, which provide a rough surface. Towards the back of the tongue, buried within the papillae, are the **taste buds** (see Chapter 4). Underneath the tongue is the **lingual artery and vein**.

Memory Jogger
The lingual artery underneath the tongue can be used to take the pulse of an animal and the lingual vein can be used as a site for venepuncture. Both these procedures should be performed on anaesthetised animals only!

- **Salivary glands** – paired structures that secrete saliva, which consists of 99% water and 1% mucus, into the oral cavity by means of ducts. Note that in the dog and the cat the saliva contains no enzymes. The glands are:
  - **zygomatic** – within the orbit, close to the eyeball
  - **sublingual** – medial to the mandible under the tongue
  - **mandibular** – caudal to the angle of the jaw
  - **parotid** – between the base of the ear and the mandibular glands.
- **Teeth** – hard structures embedded in **sockets or alveoli** in the jaw bones. Each tooth consists of a central **pulp**

cavity containing blood vessels and nerves. This is surrounded by a hard layer of **dentine**, which forms the bulk of the tooth. As the animal ages the pulp cavity shrinks and the tooth stops growing. The part of the tooth embedded in the jaw bone is known as the **root**, and here the dentine is covered in an outer layer of **cement**, consisting of fibres that anchor the tooth to the socket. Above the jaw the tooth is known as the **crown** and here the dentine is covered in a shiny white layer of hard wearing **enamel**. Once the tooth is fully grown, the only changes are due to wear.

There are four **types** of tooth, which are defined by their position in the jaw and their function.

- **Incisors (I)** – small and pointed with a single root sitting in the incisive bone and the cranial part of each mandible. Used for delicate nibbling and cutting flesh off the bone.
- **Canines (C)** – larger, pointed and curved with a single deep root. One on each corner of the upper and lower jaws. Used to hold the prey in the mouth.
- **Premolars (PM)** – also called 'cheek teeth'. Flatter surface with several pointed cusps or tubercles. May have two or three roots arranged in a triangle to provide stability in the jaw. Used to shear flesh from the bone and grind it up before swallowing.
- **Molars (M)** – also called 'cheek teeth'. Larger than premolars but similar in shape. Used for shearing and grinding flesh. There are no molars in the deciduous dentition.

   Carnassials – these are the first lower molar and the last upper premolar on each side. Carnassials are a type of cheek tooth with a similar shape but much larger. Very powerful and exert the main force of the bite. Only found in carnivores.

The number and type of teeth in each jaw is written as a **dental formula**:

Dog:	permanent	[I 3/3 C 1/1 PM 4/4 M 2/3] x 2 = 42
	deciduous	[I 3/3 C 1/1 PM 3/3] x 2 = 28
Cat:	permanent	[I 3/3 C 1/1 PM 3/2 M 1/1] x 2 = 30
	deciduous	[I 3/3 C 1/1 PM 3/2] x 2 = 26.

Table 8.1 Eruption times in the deciduous and permanent dentitions

Dentition	Tooth type	Dog Eruption time	Cat Tooth type	Eruption time
Deciduous	Incisors	3-4 weeks	All types	Begins at 2 weeks and is complete by 4 weeks
	Canines	5 weeks		
	Premolars	4-8 weeks		
Permanent	Incisors	3.5-4 months	Incisors	12 weeks
	Canines	5-6 months	Remaining teeth	Present in jaw by 6 months
	Premolars	First premolars, 4-5 months; remainder, 5-7 months		
	Molars	5-7 months		

Memory Jogger

Dental formulae are difficult to learn as they all look similar, especially when you see them on an examination paper! You may also have to remember the dental formulae of other species, such as the rabbit, rat and ferret. I am afraid there is no substitute for reciting them parrot-fashion and writing them down at every opportunity!

The dog and the cat have two sets of teeth in their lifetime:

1. **Deciduous dentition** – also called the temporary or milk teeth. These are smaller and whiter than the adult teeth. Eventually the roots dissolve and they are pushed out of the jaw by the adult teeth developing in the jaw below them. The eruption times are shown in Table 8.1.

2. **Permanent dentition** – these gradually replace the deciduous teeth. They are larger and, once in the jaw, the only change is due to wear (Table 8.1).

THE PHARYNX

This is a muscular tube lined with mucous membrane lying at the back of the oral cavity. It forms a crossover between the digestive and respiratory systems and is divided by the soft palate into the **nasopharynx** and **oropharynx** (see Chapter 7). During swallowing, food passes from the oral cavity, through the pharynx and into the oesophagus. Food is prevented from entering the larynx and trachea by the action of the **epiglottis**, which closes over the **glottis** at the entrance to the larynx. The eustachian tube from each middle ear also opens into the pharynx.

THE OESOPHAGUS

This is a simple muscular tube running from the pharynx through the neck, thoracic cavity and diaphragm to the stomach, the function of which is to convey food from the pharynx to the stomach.

It is lined with stratified squamous epithelium arranged in longitudinal folds to allow widthways expansion. Underneath are layers of circular and longitudinal smooth muscle supplied by fine networks of nerves and blood capillaries. This muscle is responsible for the generation of waves of contraction known as **peristalsis**, which push the food down towards the stomach. Food passes into the stomach within about 15–30 seconds.

THE STOMACH

In carnivores such as the dog and cat, the stomach is a C-shaped, sac-like structure with a **greater** and a **lesser curvature**. It is described as being **simple** and the type of digestion is **monogastric**.

Food enters the stomach through the **cardiac sphincter** and leaves to enter the small intestine through the **pyloric sphincter**. These are muscular structures whose function is to control the rate at which food enters and exits, and thus the amount of time it spends in the stomach.

The stomach lies predominantly on the left side of the cranial abdomen. It is easily distended with food and in the carnivore it acts as a food reservoir, enabling the animal to eat a large meal every 3–4 days and then sleep while slowly digesting it. When it is full to capacity it may occupy half of the abdominal cavity. The time taken for food to pass through the stomach - **gastric emptying time** – depends on the consistency of the food. Liquids may take as little as 30 minutes but more solid or fatty food may take more than 3 hours.

MICROSCOPIC STRUCTURE

The stomach wall is thick and arranged in deep folds or **rugae**, which flatten as the organ expands and fills with food. It consists of several layers. The inner layer of mucous membrane is made of **gastric pits** which are glands responsible for the secretion of gastric digestive juices. These comprise three types of cell, each of which contributes to the **gastric juice** mixture:

- **Parietal cells** – secrete **hydrochloric acid**, which creates an acid pH of 1.3-5. This denatures protein, facilitating digestion. It also forms part of the body's primary defence system by destroying any pathogens that may enter the stomach.
- **Chief cells** – secrete the enzyme precursor **pepsinogen**, which is converted to the active enzyme **pepsin** by the action of hydrochloric acid. Pepsin digests protein.
- **Goblet cells** – secrete large quantities of **mucus**, which lubricates the passage of food through the stomach and protects the stomach wall from autodigestion by the action of the acid and enzymes.

Memory Jogger

An enzyme is a protein that acts as a catalyst to increase the speed of a reaction. Some enzymes are produced in the form of an inactive **precursor**, which must be 'switched on' by another enzyme before it can start to work.

Beneath the gastric mucosa are layers of smooth muscle, nerve and blood capillary networks, which are responsible for the contractions of the stomach wall. Food is moved around within the stomach by **rhythmic segmentation**, which breaks up the food boluses and mixes them with the gastric juices. **Peristaltic waves** propel the food through the stomach and out through the pyloric sphincter, while **antiperistalsis** may occur during vomition.

The food resulting from the digestive process within the stomach is an acid soup-like material known as **chyme**. It contains partially digested protein but at this stage the other food groups are still undigested. Chyme is released in spurts through the pyloric sphincter into the duodenum.

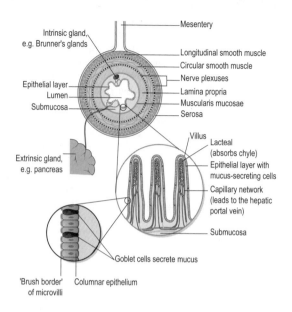

Figure 8.1 Cross-section through the intestinal wall to show the basic structure

THE SMALL INTESTINE

This is the major site of enzymic **digestion** and the subsequent **absorption** of the digested food. It is a long, relatively narrow tube divided into three parts:

- duodenum
- jejunum
- ileum.

These parts are similar in structure and it is difficult to distinguish them with the naked eye, but they do show microscopic differences related to their function.

Common structure – when looking at a cross-section of the small intestine it is possible to see four layers (Fig. 8.1):

1. **Epithelium** – this innermost layer consists of **columnar epithelium**. The outer edge of each cell has a 'brush border' of **microvilli** and the mucosa itself is arranged into numerous fingerlike projections known as **villi** (Fig. 8.1). Both of these adaptations increase the surface area available for the processes of digestion and absorption. Within the tissue of each **villus** is a branch of an arteriole and a venule, and a lymphatic capillary known as a **lacteal** (see Chapter 6). The lacteals transport digested fat globules as a liquid (known as **chyle**) to the cisterna chyli in the dorsal abdomen, where it combines with lymph. Within this epithelial layer are glands that secrete the **digestive juices** and areas of **lymphoid tissue**, which protect against infection by microorganisms.

2. **Submucosa** – a layer of connective tissue and a narrow band of smooth muscle known as the **muscularis mucosae**, which contributes to the intestinal contractions.

3. **Smooth muscle** – consists of an inner layer of **circular muscle** and an outer layer of **longitudinal muscle**. Between the layers are networks of nerve fibres that initiate and coordinate the peristaltic contractions of the muscle, propelling food along the intestine.

4. **Visceral peritoneum** – also called the **serosa** (see Chapter 2). This is a single layer of tissue that covers every abdominal organ and is continuous with the **parietal peritoneum** lining the wall of the abdominal cavity. The **mesentery** of each organ is a double layer of peritoneum, linking the visceral and parietal peritoneum, which suspends the organs in place within the peritoneal cavity. Some mesenteries are short while others are long, allowing the organs to be relatively mobile. Each mesentery is named according to the organ to which is it attached, e.g. mesoileum (see Chapter 2).

DUODENUM

This is a U-shaped loop of intestine running from the pyloric sphincter to its junction with the jejunum. It is held in a fixed position close to the roof of the dorsal abdomen by a short **mesoduodenum**. The **pancreas** lies within the loop of the duodenum and pours its exocrine secretions into the lumen by two **pancreatic ducts**. The **common bile duct** leading from the gall bladder, which lies between the lobes of the liver, also opens into the duodenum a short distance from the pyloric sphincter. Within the duodenal mucosa are **Brunner's glands**, which secrete a cocktail of digestive enzymes known collectively as **succus entericus**.

JEJUNUM AND ILEUM

Together, these form a very mobile tube, which as it has a long **mesojejunum** and **mesoileum**, is able to take up any unoccupied space in the abdomen. The junction between the two parts is difficult to distinguish. The ileum terminates at the junction of the caecum and ascending colon, known as the **ileocaecal junction**. Within the mucosa are the **crypts of Lieberkühn**, which secrete a cocktail of digestive enzymes.

THE LARGE INTESTINE

This is described as 'large' because most of the tube has a larger diameter than that of the small intestine. Within this part of the digestive system, water and electrolytes are resorbed from the material remaining after the digestive process, and mucus is added to lubricate the faecal mass. Bacteria flourish within the faeces. They are responsible for the breakdown of any remaining protein and contribute to the odour of faeces.

The large intestine consists of the:
* caecum
* colon
* rectum
* anal canal.

The basic structure is similar to that of the small intestine but there are no villi or digestive glands. However, there are numerous goblet cells, which produce mucus.
* **Caecum** – a short, blind-ending sac found at the **ileocaecal junction**. In the carnivore this has very little function (see Chapter 13).
* **Colon** – divided into the **ascending, transverse** and **descending colon** according to which direction the tube is

running; for example, the ascending colon runs cranially. The mesocolon is short and holds the colon in a fixed position.

- **Rectum** – the area of the colon that lies within the pelvic cavity and terminates at the **anal canal**. The most cranial part is covered with peritoneum but deeper into the cavity it becomes surrounded by connective tissue and muscles, which attach it to the root of the tail.

- **Anal canal** – a short tube ending in the **anal sphincter**. The lumen is lined with deep folds of mucous membrane, enabling widthways expansion as the faecal mass passes through. The anal sphincter consists of an **internal ring** of circular smooth muscle (under involuntary control) surrounded by an **external ring** of striated muscle (under voluntary control). The sphincter is normally closed but it relaxes as the faecal mass moves through the pelvic cavity, pushed by **mass movements**; these are a larger and slower form of peristalsis. As the mass reaches the anal canal, **abdominal contractions** aid expulsion of the faeces. Just proximal to the anal sphincter are a pair of **anal sacs**. These glands, lying in the '20 to 4' position, produce a secretion with an offensive smell, used as a territorial marker.

ACCESSORY STRUCTURES

These are not part of the digestive tract but they contribute to the process of digestion and absorption.

PANCREAS

This gland is extrinsic to the digestive system; i.e. it lies outside the tract within the mesoduodenum. It is pale pink and lobulated, and is classed as a **mixed gland** because it has both endocrine and exocrine parts:

- **Endocrine** part – the **Islets of Langerhans** secrete the hormones insulin, glucagon and somatostatin, all involved in the control of blood glucose (see Chapter 5).
- **Exocrine** part – secretes digestive enzymes and bicarbonate into the lumen of the duodenum via the two pancreatic ducts.

GALL BLADDER

This is a small sac lying between the lobes of the liver. It collects bile produced by the liver and empties it into the lumen of the duodenum through the **common bile duct**. Bile is a liquid containing **bile salts**, which are used to emulsify fats during digestion. Bile is stained yellow by the pigment **bilirubin**, formed during the breakdown of old red blood cells.

LIVER

This is the largest gland in the body and lies in the cranial abdomen close to the caudal surface of the diaphragm. It can be thought of as the 'factory' of the body and it has many vital **functions**:

- Carbohydrate metabolism – surplus glucose is stored as glycogen, which is released when extra energy is needed.
- Protein metabolism – production of plasma proteins.
- Fat metabolism – formation of lipids. Fatty acids are a source of energy.
- Formation of urea from ammonia, which is the breakdown product of protein metabolism. Urea is excreted by the kidneys.
- Formation of bile, which contains bilirubin from the breakdown of old red blood cells.
- Destruction of red blood cells.
- Formation of new red blood cells – occurs only in the fetus.
- Storage of the fat-soluble vitamins A, D, E and K. Some water-soluble vitamins may also be stored.
- Storage of iron.
- Production of heat – involved in thermoregulation.
- Detoxification of some substances, such as alcohol.
- Detoxification and conjugation of steroid hormones.

The liver is a deep-red organ divided into several **lobes**. In the centre, on the abdominal side is the **falciform ligament**, which is the remains of the fetal umbilical cord. The cranial surface is convex and conforms to the shape of the diaphragm while the caudal surface is concave and is closely associated with the stomach and right kidney.

Blood supply

Arterial blood reaches the liver in the **hepatic artery** and venous blood leaves in the **hepatic vein**. The products of digestion are carried from the small intestine to the liver in the **hepatic portal vein** (see Chapter 6).

Microscopic structure

The main cells of the liver are known as **hepatocytes** and they carry out all the functions of the liver. They are arranged in series of hexagonal **lobules**, at each corner of which is a branch of the **hepatic artery** and a branch of the **hepatic portal vein**. Blood from these flows across the lobule to drain into the **central vein** in the middle of the lobule, and eventually out of the liver in the **hepatic vein**. Bile formed by the hepatocytes flows through a system of **bile canaliculi**, which drain into the bile ducts and eventually into the **gall bladder**; here it is stored until needed for digestion.

DIGESTION

Digestion is the process by which food taken into the body is broken down into soluble units ready for absorption. Food consists of proteins, carbohydrates and fats, which are broken down by the action of digestive enzymes as follows:

- protein → polypeptides → peptides → amino acids
- carbohydrates → polysaccharides → disaccharides/monosaccharides
- fats (lipids) → triglycerides → monoglycerides/fatty acids.

Digestion in the carnivore takes place in the stomach and small intestine; there is no digestion within the oral cavity.

Memory Jogger

The structure of enzymes is such that they are able to act only on a specific substrate, and they are named according to that substrate. For example, lipases act on lipids, maltase acts on maltose, and aminopeptidase acts on peptides to produce amino acids. This makes it much easier to work out and remember which reaction is affected.

STOMACH

As food passes through the cardiac sphincter the walls of the stomach secrete the hormone **gastrin** (see Chapter 5). This stimulates the secretion of **gastric juices** from the gastric pits within the gastric mucosa. Gastric juices contain:

- **Mucus** – secreted by goblet cells. Lubricates the food and protects against autodigestion by the digestive enzymes.
- **Hydrochloric acid (HCl)** – secreted by parietal cells. Denatures protein, facilitating digestion. Converts pepsinogen to the active pepsin.
- **Pepsinogen** – secreted by chief cells. Precursor of pepsin.

The reaction occurring in the stomach is:

Pepsinogen + hydrochloric acid = pepsin
Pepsin + protein = peptides – a process known as hydrolysis.

The average pH in the stomach is 1.3–5, which is the ideal environment for this form of protein digestion. Food is converted into liquid **chyme**, which is 'squirted' through the pyloric sphincter into the duodenum.

SMALL INTESTINE

Secretion of digestive juices within the small intestine is controlled by:

- Passage of food through the pyloric sphincter, which stimulates the walls of the small intestine to secrete the hormone **secretin** (see Chapter 5). This initiates the production of **digestive enzymes** from the pancreas.
- Passage of food along the intestine, which stimulates the walls of the duodenum and jejunum to secrete **cholecystokinin**. This initiates contraction of the gall bladder and the release of bile.
- Parasympathetic branch of the autonomic nervous system (see Chapter 4).

There are three sources of digestive juice:

- **Pancreatic secretions** produced by the exocrine glands. These contain:
    - **Bicarbonate** – neutralises the effect of acid from the stomach.
    - **Enzymes and their precursors** – if the enzymes were in the active form they would autodigest the pancreas. The

major precursor is **trypsinogen**, which is 'switched on' to form **trypsin** by another enzyme – **enterokinase** – from Brunner's glands in the duodenum. Trypsin then switches on the other precursors. The enzymes in the pancreatic secretions are:

- **Proteases** – act on proteins and peptides, e.g. trypsin: Protein + trypsin = polypeptides + peptides.
- **Lipases** – act on fats (lipids) and are activated by bile salts: Fats + lipase = fatty acids + monoglycerides.
- **Amylases** – act on carbohydrates – mainly starch: Starch + amylase = maltose (disaccharide).

- **Bile secretions** – produced by the liver and stored in the gall bladder. Contains bile salts, which emulsify fats into small globules creating a larger surface area for the action of the digestive enzymes.

- **Intestinal secretions** – produced by the:
  - **crypts of Lieberkühn** in the jejunum and ileum
  - **Brunner's glands** in the duodenum – these secretions are known as **succus entericus**.

The secretions contain several enzymes:

- **enterokinase**: enterokinase + trypsinogen = trypsin – this switches on the other enzymes
- **aminopeptidase**: peptides + aminopeptidase = amino acids
- **lipase**: lipase + fats = fatty acids + monoglycerides
- **maltase**: maltase + maltose = glucose
- **sucrase**: sucrase + sucrose = glucose + fructose
- **lactase**: lactase + lactose = glucose + galactose.

The result of digestion is to produce amino acids; monosaccharides in the form of glucose, fructose and galactose; fatty acids; and glycerol. These molecules are all small enough to be able to pass through the epithelium of the small intestine.

Memory Jogger

Let's follow **protein** through the digestive process.

· In the stomach – HCl denatures the protein and converts pepsinogen to pepsin:

protein + pepsin = peptides

· In the small intestine - enterokinase converts trypsinogen to trypsin:

protein + trypsin = peptides

peptides + aminopeptidase = amino acids.

Memory Jogger

Let's follow **carbohydrate** through the digestive process.

· Amylase, maltase, sucrase and lactase are all present in the intestinal digestive juices:

starch + amylase = maltose

maltose + maltase = glucose

sucrose + sucrase = glucose + fructose

lactose + lactase = glucose + galactose.

Memory Jogger

Let's follow **fat** through the digestive process.

· Bile salts emulsify fat particles, facilitating digestion.

· Pancreatic juice and succus entericus both contain lipase:

fat + lipase = fatty acids and monoglycerides

ABSORPTION

The products of the enzymic digestive process are absorbed through the thin epithelial lining covering the villi of the small intestine. They pass into the blood capillaries and lacteals within the tissue of each villus:

- Amino acids and the monosaccharides glucose, fructose and galactose enter the blood capillaries and are carried to the liver by the **hepatic portal vein** (see Chapter 6).

- Fatty acids and monoglycerides enter the **lacteals**, forming a milky liquid known as **chyle**. Chyle is carried to the cisterna chyli, where it combines with lymph and drains into the thoracic duct. This eventually mixes with the blood in the right atrium of the heart (see Chapter 6).

After absorption, the digestive products are transported around the body to the tissues, where they are metabolised. This occurs in most cells, although the liver plays a significant part.

METABOLISM

Metabolism is the process in which the soluble units resulting from digestion are used by the cells to produce energy. There are two types of metabolic reaction:

- **anabolic** – reactions in which materials are formed, requiring the use of energy, e.g.

    oxygen + haemoglobin + energy = oxyhaemoglobin

- **catabolic** – reactions in which food materials are broken down into smaller units with the release of energy, e.g.

    starch = maltose + energy.

CARBOHYDRATE METABOLISM

Most carbohydrate is absorbed as glucose. Glucose is carried by the blood to the cells, where it is used to provide energy. Excess glucose is carried to the liver, where it is stored as **glycogen** – a process known as **glycogenesis**. These two processes are controlled by the hormone **insulin** secreted by the pancreas (see Chapter 6), the main function of which is to lower the blood glucose level.

If the blood glucose level falls, the stored glycogen is broken down into glucose, which is released into the blood for use by the cells – a process known as **glycogenolysis**. This is controlled by the hormone **glucagon** from the pancreas (see Chapter 6), the main function of which is to raise the blood glucose level.

PROTEIN METABOLISM

Proteins are absorbed as amino acids and are needed for growth and repair of tissues and synthesis of other proteins by the liver. They are also used for the production of energy; this results in the formation of ammonia, which is converted to urea and excreted in the urine by the kidneys. Excess amino acids are converted to urea – a process known as **deamination** and excreted, while others may be converted into more useful types of amino acid by a process known as **transamination**.

FAT METABOLISM

In the liver fats are converted into cholesterol and phospho-lipids for the formation of cell membranes and bile salts. If an animal is starved and there is no glucose available, the liver uses fat to release energy. As a by-product of this, **ketone bodies** are produced, which accumulate in the blood and urine – high levels can be fatal. If an animal is overweight, excess fat is stored in deposits around the body, giving rise to the typi-cal appearance of an obese animal.

MULTIPLE CHOICE

Now use these multiple choice questions to test your under-standing of this chapter.

1. The carnassial tooth in the lower jaw of the dog is:

a. the first molar ○

b. the second molar ○

c. the first premolar ○

d. the fourth premolar. ○

2. The dental formula for the deciduous dentition of the cat is:

a. [I 3/3 C1/1 PM 4/4 M2/3] x 2 = 42 ○

b. [I 3/3 C1/1 PM3/3] x 2 = 28 ○

c. [I 3/3 c1/1 PM 3/2 M 1/1] x 2 = 30 ○

d. [I 3/3 C1/1 PM 3/2] x 2 = 26. ○

3. The structure linking the stomach to the duodenum is the:

a. ileocaecal junction ○

b. cardiac sphincter ○

c. pyloric sphincter ○

d. common bile duct. ○

4. The partially digested material leaving the stomach is:

a. chyle and is alkaline ○

b. chyme and is neutral ○

c. chyme and is acidic ○

d. food and is alkaline. ○

5. The action of the enzyme lipase is to convert:

a. proteins to peptides

b. fats to fatty acids and monoglycerides. ○

c. lactose to glucose and galactose ○

d. starch to maltose. ○

6. Which of the following is NOT a function of the liver?

a. formation of bile from the breakdown of old red blood
cells ○

b. storage of iron ○

c. regulation of the percentage of water in the urine ○

d. detoxification of steroid hormones. ○

THE ANSWERS ARE:

1 a, 2 d, 3 c, 4 c, 5 b, 6 c.

9
The Urinary System

The urinary system is often thought to be one of the most difficult systems to grasp. However, take it slowly, step by step, make sure you understand the basic physiological processes that occur within the kidney tubules, and you will find that it is not as complicated as you first thought! An understanding of kidney function is essential if you are to understand why the symptoms of chronic and acute renal failure occur.

The urinary system, lying within the abdominal and pelvic cavities, is anatomically linked with the reproductive or genital system and together they may be referred to as the urinogenital system. In the male, urine is conveyed out of the body in the urethra, which runs through the penis, whereas in the female the urethra conveys urine to the junction of the vagina and vestibule and it flows out of the body via the vestibule and vulva.

The **functions** of the urinary system are to:

- regulate the chemical composition and volume of the body fluids, this is known as **osmoregulation** and is a vital part of homeostasis
- remove waste products and excess water from the body – this is known as **excretion**
- secrete the hormone **erythropoietin**, which stimulates the production of red blood cells from the bone marrow (see Chapter 6).

Memory Jogger

Homeostasis is the way in which the internal environment of the body is kept in a state of equilibrium, so that all the body processes can work effectively. It involves osmoregulation, thermoregulation, respiration, buffers within the blood and excretion. Maintenance of homeostasis depends on information being sent to the brain from the nervous and endocrine systems.

The **parts** of the system are:

- kidneys – a pair
- ureters – a pair
- bladder
- urethra.

THE KIDNEY

- There is a **pair** of kidneys lying one on either side of the midline just ventral to the lumbar vertebrae.
- They are closely related to the caudal vena cava and aorta, and lie caudal to the adrenal glands, and in the female they are cranial to the ovaries. The left kidney is slightly caudal to the right because developmentally it is displaced by the stomach.
- Each kidney lies between the roof of the abdominal cavity and the parietal peritoneum and is described as being **retroperitoneal**. There is no suspensory mesentery.
- The **size** of a normal kidney approximates to two and a half lumbar vertebrae when viewed on a radiograph.
- The normal **colour** is deep browny-red, but as the kidney filters the blood the colour may be changed by disease or any chemicals carried in the blood.
- The normal **shape** is that of a kidney bean. The indented area is known as the **hilus**.
- If you examine the cut surface of a kidney it is possible to identify the following layers:
  - outer protective **capsule** – made of dense connective tissue and often surrounded by fat
  - **cortex** – dark red in colour. Contains the **glomeruli** and the **convoluted tubules** of the nephrons
  - **medulla** – slightly paler red. Triangular areas known as the **pyramids** may be distinguishable; these are the sites of the **collecting ducts**. Also contains the **loops of Henle**
  - **pelvis** – almost white because of the high proportion of fibrous connective tissue. This is a basin-shaped area that collects urine formed by the nephrons
  - **ureter** – connects with the kidney at the hilus and drains urine from the pelvis
- Blood reaches the kidney from the aorta via a single **renal artery**. This divides into several **interlobar arteries**, which then divide into i**nterlobular arteries**, giving off branches to the **glomeruli**. Blood returns in the **interlobular veins**, which flow into the **interlobar veins** and out of the kidney through the single **renal vein**. The blood supply to the kidney takes up 20% of cardiac output.

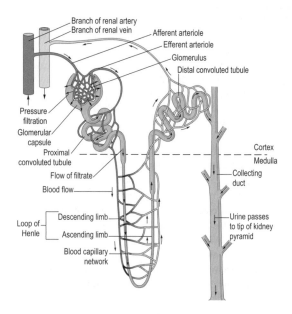

Figure 9.1 A renal nephron

MICROSCOPIC STRUCTURE

The functional unit of the kidney is the **nephron** (Fig. 9.1) Each kidney consists of about one million nephrons packed tightly into the organ. The space between the nephrons is filled with interstitial tissue and blood capillaries.

Each nephron is divided into several parts, each of which contributes to the formation of urine. The parts of the nephron and their location within the layers of the kidney are shown in Table 9.1.

- **Glomerular capsule** – a hollow, cup-shaped structure, also called **Bowman's capsule**, enclosing a knot of blood capillaries called the **glomerulus**. The glomerular capsule and the glomerulus form the **renal corpuscle** or the **Malpighian corpuscle**. The inner layer of the capsule forms a **base-**

Table 9.1 Parts of the renal nephron

Part of nephron	Site within the kidney
Glomerular capsule	Cortex
Proximal convoluted tubule	Cortex
Loop of Henle	Medulla
Distal convoluted tubule	Cortex
Collecting duct	Medulla – within the pyramids

ment membrane, which is perforated by minute pores. This is closely applied to the endothelium of the glomerular capillaries and acts as a selective filter that allows fluid and small molecules to flow through but holds back the passage of larger molecules – a process known as **ultra-filtration**.

- **Proximal convoluted tubule** – connects to the glomerular capsule by a short neck. Lined with simple cuboidal or columnar epithelium, the inner surface of which is lined with fine microvilli, forming a brush border to increase the surface area available for reabsorption.
- **Loop of Henle** – a U-shaped tube that extends into the medulla. Comprises a descending and an ascending part. Both are lined with squamous epithelium but this is thicker in the ascending part.
- **Distal convoluted tubule** – lies in the cortex and is lined with cuboidal epithelium without a brush border.
- **Collecting duct** – collects urine from several nephrons. Collections of ducts accumulate in the pyramids. The lining changes from cuboidal to columnar epithelium as it gets nearer to the pyramids.

TUBULAR FUNCTION – THE FORMATION OF URINE

Each section of the renal tubule plays a different part in the formation of urine, which is achieved by a series of additions and subtractions to and from the original glomerular filtrate. The resulting urine is very different from the filtrate in terms of concentration and volume – for every 100 litres of filtrate only 1 litre is excreted as urine, or 1% of the original filtrate.

Memory Jogger

To understand the processes occurring within the renal tubules it is important to remember the meaning of the following terms:

Osmosis – the passage of water across a semipermeable membrane from a weaker to a stronger solution. This is a passive process.

Diffusion – the passage of a substance from an area of high concentration to an area of low concentration. This is a passive process.

Reabsorption – the passage of chemical substances from the lumen of the renal tubules into the renal capillaries, and so back into the body. This is an active process that requires the expenditure of energy.

Secretion – the passage of chemical substances from the renal capillaries into the lumen of the renal tubules, and so out of the body in the urine. This is an active process that requires the expenditure of energy.

Blood carrying oxygen and waste materials enters the kidney via the renal artery and is distributed to the glomeruli within the glomerular capsules.

- **Glomerular capsule** – blood pressure within each glomerulus is high because the blood comes directly from the renal artery and the aorta, which carry blood under pressure, and because the walls of the efferent arteriole of the glomerulus are able to constrict under the influence of the hormone **renin**.

High pressure forces fluid and small molecules out through the pores of the basement membrane into the lumen of the glomerular capsule. This process of **ultrafiltration** results in the formation of a fluid known as the **glomerular filtrate** or **primitive urine**. It is very dilute and consists of 99% water and 1% chemical solutes and is isotonic with plasma (see Chapter 2).

- **Proximal convoluted tubule** – the functions of this part of the tubule are:

  - reabsorption of glucose, water and sodium (Na+) from the filtrate – normal urine leaving the bladder contains no glucose

  - secretion of toxins and certain drugs such as penicillin and its derivatives

  - concentration of nitrogenous waste – mainly urea produced as a result of protein metabolism. The level of urea becomes more concentrated as water is resorbed.

The glomerular filtrate leaving this part of the tubule has a pH of 7.4, is isotonic with plasma, and has lost 65% of its original water content and 80% of its original chemical solutes.

- **Loop of Henle** – the filtrate passes first into the descending loop and then into the ascending loop (Fig. 9.1). Its function is to concentrate or dilute the filtrate according to the status of the blood plasma and the rest of the extracellular fluid (ECF). This occurs in two stages:
  - in the **descending loop** – water is drawn out of the filtrate by Na+ ions in the surrounding medullary tissue and is resorbed by the capillaries
  - in the **ascending loop** – Na+ is pumped out of the filtrate into the medullary tissue.

Memory Jogger

The loop of Henle works on the principle of a countercurrent multiplier system. To understand this, imagine that the flow of filtrate through the loop stops for a moment.

· Na+ and Cl- are pumped out of the **ascending loop** into the tissue of the surrounding medulla. Normally water would follow Na+ by osmosis but the walls of the ascending loop are impermeable to water, so this does not happen.

· The walls of the **descending loop** are permeable to water, so water is drawn out by osmosis as a result of the high concentration of Na+ ions in the medullary tissue pumped out of the ascending limb.

Now imagine that the filtrate begins to flow again and return to the description in the text.

The resulting filtrate, now referred to as urine, is more concentrated and is reduced in volume. The urine is at its greatest concentration at the tip of the loop of Henle.

- **Distal convoluted tubule** – the function of this is to make final adjustments to the chemical make-up of the urine in response to the status of the blood plasma and the ECF. This is under the control of the hormone **aldosterone** and is achieved by:
  - reabsorption of Na+ ions
  - excretion of K+ ions
  - regulation of the **acid–base balance** or pH of the blood by the excretion of H+ ions. Normal pH of the blood is 7.4.

  For every Na+ ion reabsorbed, one K+ or H+ is excreted.

In this part of the renal tubule water is not reabsorbed in any great quantity.

- **Collecting duct** – each collecting duct receives urine from several tubules. The collecting ducts accumulate in the **pyramid** areas of the kidney and urine flows into the renal **pelvis**. The function of the collecting duct is to make final adjustments to the water content of the urine. This change occurs by altering the permeability of the duct walls to water under the control of **antidiuretic hormone or ADH**.

 Memory Jogger

An **electrolyte** is a substance that breaks up into ions when dissolved in water.

An **ion** is a charged particle.

A **cation** is a positively charged particle; examples are Na+ (sodium) and K+ (potassium).

An **anion** is a negatively charged particle; examples are Cl– (chloride) and HCO_3– (bicarbonate).

Memory Jogger

The pH scale is a measure of the hydrogen (H+) ion concentration in a solution.

· When the level of H+ ions is high the solution is acid and the pH will be between 7 and 1.

· When the level of H+ ions is low the solution is alkaline and the pH will be between 7 and 14.

· Neutral pH is 7.

OSMOREGULATION

'Osmoregulation' is the name given to the control of water balance and the regulation of the electrolytes within the body fluids by the formation and excretion of urine. The final composition of urine is based on the status of the blood plasma and the ECF at the time. Osmoregulation is one of the vital homeostatic mechanisms necessary to ensure that the body is able to function normally.

Osmoregulation occurs in two ways:

- Control of the amount of **water** lost from the body. This affects the volume of the fluid compartments (see Chapter 2).
- Control of the amount of **salt** or sodium (Na+) lost from the body. This affects the osmotic pressure of the body fluids (see Chapter 2).

Table 9.2 Factors involved in osmoregulation

Factor	Function
Renin	Produced by the renal glomeruli in response to low arterial blood pressure
Angiotensinogen	Plasma protein converted to active angiotensin by the action of renin
Angiotensin	Causes vasoconstriction and stimulates the secretion of aldosterone from the adrenal cortex
Aldosterone	Secreted by the cortex of the adrenal gland (see Chapter 5) in response to the presence of angiotensin in the blood. Acts on the distal convoluted tubules of the renal nephron to control the reabsorption of Na+ ions and the acid-base balance
Antidiuretic hormone – ADH or vasopressin	Secreted by the posterior pituitary gland (see Chapter 5). Acts on the collecting ducts of the renal nephrons. Alters the permeability of the duct walls to the passage of water
Baroreceptors	Found within the walls of blood vessels. Monitor levels of arterial blood pressure
Osmoreceptors	Found within the hypothalamus of the brain. Monitor the osmotic pressure of the blood plasma and influence the secretion of ADH from the posterior pituitary gland

Table 9.2 lists the factors involved in osmoregulation.

CONTROL OF WATER IN THE BODY

Water is lost from the body mainly in the faeces, urine, sweat and respiration, and smaller amounts are lost in tears and vaginal discharges. It is replaced by water in food and drink. If water loss is excessive, which may occur in cases of diarrhoea and vomiting, the volume of fluid in the body compartments (particularly the blood plasma) falls, and the animal is said to be **dehydrated**. The regulatory mechanisms then begin to work.

Memory Jogger
Blood pressure – the pressure exerted by the blood on the inner walls of the blood vessels. Detected by baroreceptors.
Osmotic pressure – the pressure needed to prevent osmosis from occurring. Depends on the number of undissolved particles and ions in a solution. Detected by osmoreceptors.

The regulation of water levels in the body follows a logical step-by-step process. Let us follow one such sequence.

Suppose that the animal is dehydrated:

1. Loss of water results in a fall in the volume of the blood plasma.
2. The fall in volume results in a fall in blood pressure – this is described as **hypotension**.
3. Low blood pressure is detected by **baroreceptors** (Table 9.2) and the information is relayed to the posterior pituitary gland at the base of the brain (see Chapter 5).
4. The posterior pituitary gland secretes **antidiuretic hormone (ADH)**.
5. ADH increases the permeability of the walls of the collecting ducts of the renal nephrons to water.
6. Water is reabsorbed from the urine in the collecting ducts into the blood capillaries and so back into the circulation.
7. Plasma volume increases and blood pressure returns to normal.
8. The output of urine is reduced – this is described as **oliguria**.
9. At the same time, a fall in blood volume causes a rise in the **osmotic pressure** of the Na+ ions in the blood.
10. The rise in osmotic pressure is detected by the **osmoreceptors** (Table 9.2). The osmoreceptors stimulate the **thirst centre** of the brain and the animal feels the need to drink. Excessive thirst is described as **polydipsia**.
11. The intake of water increases the blood volume.
12. Thus, blood pressure rises to the normal level and osmotic pressure falls.

From this you can deduce that a dehydrated animal may show hypotension, oliguria and polydipsia.

Now try to work out for yourself the sequence that takes place if the body retains water so that blood pressure rises – hypertension.

CONTROL OF SALT LEVELS IN THE BODY

Salt or sodium chloride (NaCl) is taken into the body in food and is lost in urine, faeces and sweat. Within the body, salt is found in some form in all the fluid compartments and it plays an important part in determining the osmotic pressure of the fluids. If the balance of salt is altered by the ingestion of excessive quantities or by excessive loss, as in vomiting and diarrhoea, regulatory mechanisms begin to work.

The regulation of salt levels in the body follows a logical step-by-step process. Let us follow one such sequence.

Suppose the animal has lost excessive amounts of salt from the body:

1. Low levels of Na+ ions in the blood result in a fall in the osmotic pressure of the plasma.
2. The fall in osmotic pressure results in fluid loss from the plasma into the extracellular fluid.
3. Fluid loss from the plasma results in a fall in blood volume and a consequent fall in blood pressure – **hypotension**.
4. This fall in blood pressure stimulates the production of **renin** (Table 9.2) from the glomeruli.
5. Renin acts as a catalyst in the conversion of the plasma protein **angiotensinogen** to **angiotensin**.
6. Angiotensin constricts the blood vessels, which helps to raise blood pressure.
7. **Angiotensin** also stimulates the thirst centre, causing the animal to drink, increasing fluid volume.
8. Angiotensin also stimulates the release of the hormone **aldosterone** from the cortex of the adrenal gland (see Chapter 5).
9. Aldosterone acts on the distal convoluted tubules of the renal nephrons, increasing the reabsorption of Na+ ions from the urine back into the blood capillaries.
10. Increased levels of Na+ in the blood raise the osmotic pressure.
11. Fluid is drawn into the blood plasma by osmosis.
12. The blood volume increases and blood pressure returns to normal.

An animal that has lost excessive amounts of salt will be **hypotensive** and, because salt is involved in a wide range of reactions in the body, it may show many other symptoms, such as muscle cramping. In fact salt is usually lost with water, so that symptoms include those associated with dehydration.

Now try to work out for yourself the sequence that takes place if the animal has eaten excessive amounts of salt.

EXCRETION

Excretion is the removal from the body of waste products formed as a result of metabolic processes within the cells and tissues. These waste products are either potentially harmful to the body or are surplus to requirements and pass out of the body in the urine.

The waste products include:

- **Water** – taken in with food and drink and excreted in varying amounts depending on the volume of the body fluids. Controlled by osmoregulation.

- **Inorganic ions** – taken into the body in food and drink and excreted in varying amounts depending on the osmotic pressure of the body fluids. Controlled by osmoregulation.

- **Nitrogenous waste products** – formed during protein metabolism. Protein is taken into the body in food and broken down into amino acids by the process of digestion (see Chapter 8). Amino acids are carried to the liver and other tissues, where they are used to build up the proteins of the body. Surplus amino acids cannot be stored by the liver and are broken down by a process of **deamination**, which results in ammonia as a by-product. Ammonia is toxic to all tissues, particularly those of the nervous system, and must be excreted. In a series of processes known as the **ornithine cycle**, ammonia is combined with carbon dioxide to form **urea**; this is transported from the liver to the kidneys, where it is excreted in the urine.

- **Detoxification products** – these include hormones, certain drugs and many poisons that are inactivated by the liver and excreted in the urine.

Memory Jogger

Normal urine contains only water, salts and urea!

Urine formed by the renal nephrons leaves each kidney and flows into the remainder of the urinary tract.

URETER

Each ureter is a thin tube that leaves the kidney from an area known as the **hilus** and carries urine to the bladder. The tube is lined with transitional epithelium, under which runs a layer of smooth muscle whose rhythmic contractions force urine along the tube by peristalsis. It is suspended in a layer of peritoneum known as the **mesoureter**. The ureter enters the bladder, close to the neck at the **trigone**.

BLADDER

This is a blind-ended, pear-shaped, hollow organ whose function is to store urine before micturition. It lies in the midline with the rounded end pointing cranially and the narrow end or **neck** pointing caudally. When empty, the bladder lies almost entirely within the pelvic cavity but as it fills with urine it extends into the caudal abdominal cavity and may touch the ventral abdominal wall.

The bladder is lined with **transitional epithelium**, which allows expansion as it fills with urine. Beneath this are layers of elastic tissue and smooth muscle and an outer layer of peritoneum that covers only the cranial end, lying in the abdominal cavity.

Each ureter enters the bladder obliquely in an area close to the neck known as the **trigone**. Here, the ureter runs under the bladder mucosa, preventing the backflow of urine.

The caudal end is extended into the **neck** and ends as the **bladder sphincter**. This muscular structure, which controls the flow of urine out of the bladder, consists of an inner ring of smooth muscle under involuntary control and an outer ring of striated muscle under voluntary or conscious control.

URETHRA

This carries urine from the bladder sphincter caudally through the pelvic cavity to the outside of the body. In the male it is also used to introduce sperm from the testes into the female reproductive tract.

There is a difference in anatomy between the female and the male.

- **Female** – the urethra is a short tube that opens into the ventral floor of the reproductive tract at the junction of the vagina and vestibule (see Chapter 10) at a point known as the **external urethral orifice**.
- **Male** – there is a difference in anatomy between the dog and the tomcat.

  - **Dog** – as the urethra leaves the bladder it is penetrated by two openings from the **deferent ducts** from the testes and one from the **prostate gland**, which surrounds the urethra (see Chapter 10). From this point the urethra conveys both urine and semen to the outside. The urethra then curves ventrally over the ischial arch, leaving the pelvic cavity and running cranially within the erectile tissue of the penis.

  - **Tomcat** – there is a longer length of tube between the bladder sphincter and the opening of the prostate gland, known as the **preprostatic urethra**. As in the dog, there are also two openings from the deferent ducts. The urethra runs caudally through the pelvic cavity. Close to the tip it is penetrated by the openings from a pair of **bulbourethral glands** and surrounded by the erectile tissue of the penis. The penis of the tomcat points backwards and does not have the additional length of penile urethra outside the pelvic cavity.

MICTURITION

Micturition is the act of expelling urine from the bladder and is normally a reflex activity. It occurs in the following way:

1. The bladder becomes distended with urine.
2. Distension of the smooth muscle in the bladder walls stimulates stretch receptors within the muscle.
3. Information from the stretch receptors is carried to the spinal cord by sensory nerves.

Table 9.3 Urinalysis – Adapted from *Introduction to Veterinary Anatomy and Physiology* (Aspinall and O'Reilly, 2004)

Clinical parameter	Normal value	Comments
Daily volume	*Dog:* 20–100 ml/kg body weight *Cat:* 10–12 ml/kg body weight	Polyuria – increased volume of urine Oliguria – reduced volume of urine Anuria – absence of urine
Appearance	Clear, yellow, characteristic smell	Tomcat urine has an unpleasant, strong smell. Old samples smell ammoniacal
pH	5–7	Carnivorous diet produces acid urine. Herbivorous diet produces alkaline urine
Specific gravity	*Dog:* 1.016–1.060 *Cat:* 1.020–1.040	Reflects the concentration of urine. Exercise, high environmental temperatures and dehydration will cause a rise in specific gravity
Protein	None	Proteinuria – presence of protein. May indicate damage to nephrons, chronic renal failure, inflammation of the urinary tract
Blood	None	Haematuria – presence of blood Haemoglobinuria – presence of haemoglobin. Due to rupture of red cells May indicate damage or infection of the tract
Glucose	None	Glucosuria – presence of glucose. May indicate diabetes mellitus. Levels of glucose in the filtrate exceed the renal threshold and excess is excreted in the urine
Ketones	None	Ketonuria – presence of ketones. May be accompanied by acid pH and smell of peardrops in urine and on the breath
Bile	None	Bilirubinuria – presence of bile. Indicator of some form of liver disease
Crystals and casts	In small quantities these may be considered to be normal	Crystalline or colloidal material coalesces to form a cast of the renal tubules and is flushed out by the urine. In large quantities, crystals may form calculi or uroliths and block the tract

4. Parasympathetic motor nerves from the sacral area of the spinal cord cause contraction of the smooth muscle in the bladder wall.

5. As the bladder contracts, the internal bladder sphincter, also made of smooth muscle and under involuntary control, relaxes and urine is expelled.

If it is inappropriate to micturate, the process can be controlled voluntarily. The brain overrides the reflex pathway and prevents the sphincter from relaxing. When the appropriate moment occurs, both the external and internal sphincters relax and urine is released.

URINALYSIS

Urine is formed by the ultrafiltration and consequent modification of blood plasma by its passage through the renal nephrons, and it reflects the current health status of the whole animal. As a result it is a useful diagnostic tool – analysis of urine is referred to as urinalysis.

Values and terms used in urinalysis are summarised in Table 9.3.

MULTIPLE CHOICE

Now use these multiple choice questions to test your understanding of this chapter.

1. Which one of the following is NOT a function of the kidney?

a. regulation of the chemical composition of the body fluids ○

b. acting as an endocrine gland secreting the hormone erythropoietin ○

c. detoxification of corticosteroids ○

d. excretion of water and waste products. ○

2. Which one of the following statements about the kidney is FALSE?

a. It is deep red in colour and is shaped like a kidney bean. ○

b. It is suspended from the dorsal abdominal body cavity by the mesokidney. ○

c. It measures approximately 2.5 vertebrae when examined on a radiograph. ○

d. On the cut surface it is possible to identify the cortex, medulla and pelvis. ○

3. Within the kidney the loops of Henle are found in the:

a. medulla ○

b. pelvis ○

c. cortex ○

d. capsule. ○

4. Which of the following statements is FALSE?

a. Aldosterone acts on the distal convoluted tubules of the nephron. ○

b. If the levels of sodium in the blood rise, renin will be released from the glomeruli. ○

c. Baroreceptors measure changes in blood pressure. ○

d. Antidiuretic hormone will be secreted from the posterior pituitary gland in cases of dehydration. ○

5. The internal sphincter of the bladder is made of which type of muscle?

a. skeletal ○

b. striated ○

c. cardiac ○

d. smooth. ○

6. Normal urine contains:

a. water, salts and haemoglobin ○

b. water, protein and glucose ○

c. water, salts and urea ○

d. water, salts and penicillin. ○

THE ANSWERS ARE:

1 c, 2 b, 3 a, 4 b, 5 d, 6 c.

10
The Reproductive System

Reproduction is the means by which organisms ensure the survival of their species into the next generation. We take it for granted that mammals come in two different sexes, but if you study other living things you will find that this is not universal.

There are two types of reproduction:
- **Asexual** – requires only one parent and produces offspring that are genetically identical to the parent and to each other. Occurs in less highly evolved species, such as bacteria and fungi, and in some plants and animals.
- **Sexual** – requires two parents, usually of different sexes, and involves the exchange of genetic material. It produces offspring that are genetically different from the parents and from each other.

Some organisms can reproduce by both methods, but in more highly developed species, such as the vertebrates, sexual reproduction is the only means of producing offspring.

The reproductive system is also called the urinogenital system because of its shared anatomy with the urinary system (see Chapter 9). In the female animal the reproductive system is found in both the abdominal and pelvic cavities, while in the male it lies within the pelvic cavity.

THE MALE REPRODUCTIVE TRACT

The tracts of the dog and the cat are similar; where there are differences these will be highlighted (Figs 10.1 and 10.2).

The male dog is called a **dog**; the male cat is called a **tom-cat**.

The **functions** of the male tract are to:
- produce spermatozoa (sperm) to fertilise the ovum produced by the female – **spermatogenesis**
- produce seminal fluids that aid the survival of the sperm and transport them up into the female tract

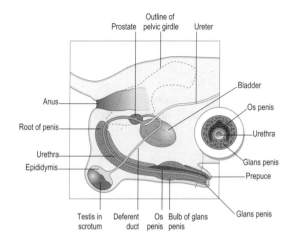

Figure 10.1 Reproductive system of the dog

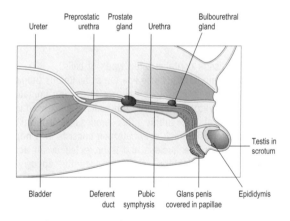

Figure 10.2 Reproductive system of the tomcat

- secrete hormones that bring about the development of the secondary sexual characteristics and affect male behaviour and spermatogenesis
- introduce sperm into the female reproductive tract.

The **parts** of the male tract are:

- testis
- epididymis
- ductus deferens
- urethra
- penis
- prostate gland – an accessory gland
- bulbourethral glands – accessory glands – seen only in the cat.

TESTIS

This is the male gonad. In the adult a pair of testes lies outside the body cavity within the **scrotum**. Externally, each testis is covered in a fibrous connective tissue capsule known as the **tunica albuginea**. Internally it consists of numerous coiled **seminiferous tubules**, which eventually unite to form the **epididymis**. This runs externally along the dorsolateral border of the testis. At the caudal extremity of the testis, the tail or **cauda epididymis** is a dilated part of the tube in which the sperm mature and are stored ready for use. The epididymis continues as the **ductus deferens**, passing out of the scrotum and entering the abdominal cavity through the **inguinal canal**.

The testicular tissue contains three types of cells:

- **Spermatogenic cells** – these line the seminiferous tubules. They divide by meiosis (see Chapter 1) to form immature tailless spermatozoa or **spermatids** which are released into the lumen of the tubule. This process is known as **spermatogenesis**. Each spermatozoon consists of a **head**, which contains the nucleus and is protected by an **acrosome cap**; a **midpiece**, which provides the energy for movement; and a long **tail**, which provides the propulsive force that enables the sperm to swim through the tubules.
- **Sertoli cells** – these line the seminiferous tubules. They secrete nutrients to aid the survival of the spermatids; they also secrete the hormone **oestrogen**.
- **Interstitial cells or the cells of Leydig** – these lie between the seminiferous tubules. They secrete **testosterone** under the control of **interstitial cell stimulating hormone** secreted by the anterior pituitary gland (see Chapter 5).

Testosterone has an effect on:

- spermatogenesis
- development of the secondary sexual characteristics, which occurs at the onset of sexual maturity or **puberty**; these include muscle development, changes in the distribution of hair, and changes in body size
- male behaviour, including aggression, territoriality and sexual behaviour.

SCROTUM

This is a relatively hairless, often pigmented external sac that in the dog lies between the thighs and in the cat lies ventral to the anus. The testes are held outside the body to provide a lower temperature; this facilitates spermatogenesis, which is inhibited at temperatures above 40°C. Internally, the scrotum is divided into two parts by a connective tissue septum. Within the walls is the **dartos muscle**, a layer of smooth muscle whose function in cold weather is to contract and pull the scrotum closer to the body, thus warming the testes.

SPERMATIC CORD

Within the scrotum, each testis is wrapped in a double layer of epithelium known as the **tunica vaginalis**, which is an evagination of the peritoneum that lines the abdominal cavity. The tunica vaginalis wraps around the structures entering and leaving the testis to form the spermatic cord. This contains the:

- spermatic or testicular artery
- spermatic or testicular vein
- spermatic nerve
- ductus deferens.

Within the tissue of the spermatic cord is the **cremaster muscle**, which in cold weather contracts in conjunction with the dartos muscle to pull the testis closer to the body.

Descent of the testis – during embryonic development each testis develops within the abdominal cavity close to the kidneys. Around the time of birth, a band of tissue or **gubernaculum**, attached at one end to the caudal end of the testis and at the other to the inside of the scrotal sac, contracts and gradually pulls the testis caudally through the abdomen towards the scrotum. The testis leaves the abdomen through the **inguinal canal**, a split in the abdominal wall in the area of the groin, and becomes wrapped in a double layer of the peritoneum, which forms the **tunica vaginalis**.

The testes should be palpable within the scrotum by the age of 12 weeks in the dog and at 10–12 weeks in the tomcat. Failure of the testes to descend is described as **cryptorchidism**. This may be an inherited condition.

DUCTUS DEFERENS

This is also called the 'vas deferens' or the 'deferent duct'. There is a pair of ductus deferentia, each of which is associated with one of the testes. Each ductus deferens consists of a narrow tube leading from the epididymis to the urethra and forms part of the spermatic cord. It conducts sperm from the testis to the urethra, entering the abdominal cavity via the inguinal canal and joining the urethra at a point that is surrounded by the **prostate gland** (Figs 10.1 and 10.2).

URETHRA AND PENIS

These form a narrow tube that is shared by the urinary and reproductive systems and runs from the neck of the bladder to the outside. Its function is to convey sperm, seminal fluid and urine out of the body (see Chapter 9). There is a difference in the anatomy of the penis between the dog and the cat.

- **Dog** – the urethra leaves the neck of the bladder and runs caudally on the floor of the pelvic cavity. As it leaves the cavity and passes over the edge of the ischial arch, it is surrounded by a layer of erectile tissue known as the **corpus cavernosum penis**, and is then referred to as the penis. The penis curves cranioventrally and passes between the thighs of the dog. It is attached to the ischial arch by a pair of fibrous tissue **crura** (singular crus), which form the **root** of the penis. The distal quarter of the penis, known as the **bulb**, becomes swollen during erection, forming a hard collar around the base. The remaining part, forming the tip, is known as the **glans penis**. Within the tissue of the glans penis and lying dorsal to the urethra is the bony **os penis**. This aids insertion of the penis into the female vagina during the early stages of mating.

- **Tomcat** – the parts of the penis are similar to those of the dog, but the penis is much shorter and points caudally, the external opening lying in the perineum ventral to the anus. During erection the penis elongates and curves cranioventrally, so that the mating position is similar to that in the dog. Within the tissue of the penis *ventral* to the urethra is the **os penis**. The tip of the penis is covered with tiny **barbs**; when the penis is withdrawn from the female at the end of mating, these cause a moment of intense pain in the female that initiates a nervous and hormonal pathway, resulting in ovulation 36 hours later.

The entire relaxed penis lies within a sheath of hairy skin known as the **prepuce**. This is lined with mucous membrane and lubricating glands and, in the dog, is suspended from the ventral abdominal wall.

Memory Jogger
Cavernous erectile tissue consists of connective tissue perforated by 'caverns' or spaces lined by endothelium. It is found within the tissue of the penis of the male and within the clitoris of the female. During sexual excitement the heart rate rises, blood is pumped into the spaces under pressure and the tissue becomes engorged or erect.

Memory Jogger
To remember the position in which the os penis lies in relation to the urethra, link the words **DO**RSAL and **DO**G and therefore the words VENTRAL and CAT

ACCESSORY GLANDS
Associated with the male tract are two types of glands which secrete fluid that is referred to collectively as **seminal fluid**. The functions of seminal fluid are:
- to provide a suitable environment for the survival of sperm as they pass through the male and female tracts
- to neutralise the acidity of any urine that may remain in the male tract
- to increase the volume of the ejaculate, which helps to propel the sperm up into the female tract.

The accessory glands are the:
- **Prostate gland** – seen in the dog and the tomcat. Lies on the floor of the pelvic cavity surrounding the urethra as it leaves the bladder. In the dog it lies close to the neck of

the bladder, while in the tomcat there is a short length of urethra between the neck and the prostate gland – this is the **preprostatic urethra**. Prostatic fluid enters the urethra through multiple ducts at a point close to the entrance of the ductus deferentia.

- **Bulbourethral glands** – seen in the tomcat. Lie on either side of the urethra close to the tip of the penis, caudal to the prostate and cranial to the ischial arch.

THE FEMALE REPRODUCTIVE TRACT

The female dog is called a **bitch**; the female cat is called a **queen**.

Both the bitch and the queen are described as being **multiparous** or litter-bearing animals; thus, their reproductive tracts are adapted to hold several offspring at the same time. The tract comprises two long uterine horns with a small uterine body – this is described as being a **bicornuate** (two-horned) uterus (Fig. 10.3).

Memory Jogger
Multiparous – the animal gives birth to several offspring at the same time; examples are the dog, cat, pig, rabbit.
Uniparous – the animal gives birth to one offspring at a time; examples are the horse and humans.
Primigravid – the animal is pregnant for the first time.
Multigravid – the animal is pregnant for the second or subsequent time.

The **functions** of the female tract are:
- to produce eggs or ova for fertilisation by the male's spermatozoa
- to secrete the female reproductive hormones oestrogen and progesterone
- to provide a receptacle in which the fertilised ova can develop into the offspring for the next generation
- to provide a means of nutritional support for the developing embryo or fetus.

The **parts** of the female tract are:
- ovary
- uterine tube
- uterus – with a uterine body and a pair of uterine horns
- cervix

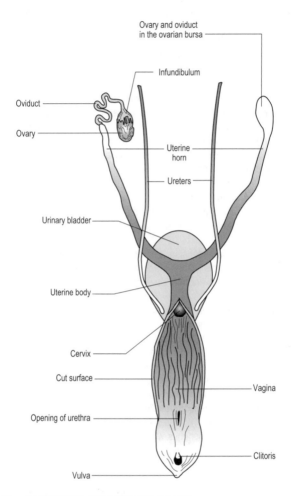

Figure 10.3 Reproductive system of the bitch and queen

- vagina
- vestibule
- vulva.

Although the mammary glands are not part of the reproductive tract, they play a vital part in reproduction.

Ovary – the female gonad. There is a pair of ovaries, one lying on each side of the dorsal abdominal cavity caudal to the kidney and the adrenal gland. Each ovary is held in position by the:

- **Ovarian ligament** – this suspensory ligament contains smooth muscle fibres, which in the pregnant animal stretch as the weight of the developing fetuses pulls the uterus down into the abdominal cavity.
- **Mesovarium** – part of the visceral peritoneum covering the ovary. Also covers the part of the **uterine tubes** and the **infundibulum**. Part of the mesovarium forms a pocket-like structure known as the **ovarian bursa**, which completely encloses the ovary.

The blood supply to the ovary is via the **ovarian artery**, which leaves the aorta in the same area as the renal artery or the testicular artery in the male (see Chapter 6).

The ovarian tissue consists of a framework of connective tissue and blood vessels within which large numbers of undifferentiated germ cells eventually develop into follicles containing ova.

Uterine tube – also called the oviduct or Fallopian tube. This narrow tube lies close to the ovary and curls over it within the mesovarium. The open end widens into a funnel-shaped **infundibulum**, which is fringed by fingerlike **fimbriae** and is able to move over the surface of the ovary to collect each ovum as it is released from the follicle. The ovum then passes down the lumen of the uterine tube. The tube is lined with ciliated columnar epithelium, which wafts the ovum down towards the **uterine horn**. It is suspended in the abdominal cavity by a layer of visceral peritoneum known as the **mesosalpinx**, which is continuous with the mesovarium.

Uterus – a Y-shaped structure lying in the midline of the caudal abdominal cavity. It comprises a small central **uterine body**, which gives off a pair of long **uterine horns**, each of which is about five times the length of the uterine body. During pregnancy the developing embryos implant at equal distances along the uterine horns so that each embryo has the maximum amount of space in which to grow.

Internally the uterus is lined by the **endometrium**, which consists of columnar epithelial cells, glandular tissue and blood capillaries. The endometrium becomes thickened during pregnancy, ready for the implantation of the placenta. Beneath it is the **myometrium**. This is made of smooth muscle fibres, which are responsible for the strong contractions that occur during parturition. The outermost layer is formed by the **mesometrium** or **broad ligament**, which is continuous with the mesovarium and the mesosalpinx and suspends the uterus in the abdomen.

Cervix – connects the uterus to the vagina. It is a thick-walled structure through which runs a narrow **cervical canal**, which allows the passage of sperm up into the uterus and dilates to let the fetuses into the birth canal during parturition. In non-pregnant animals the cervix lies within the pelvic cavity, but during pregnancy it is pulled cranially and ventrally over the pelvic brim by the weight of the developing fetuses in the uterine horns.

Vagina – extends from the cervix to the **external urethral orifice**, which is the point at which the urethra joins the reproductive tract. It lies entirely in the pelvic cavity. The internal surface of the vagina consists of longitudinal folds, which allow widthways expansion during parturition. In the bitch the lining of stratified squamous epithelium undergoes changes in response to the reproductive hormones of the oestrous cycle. Daily vaginal smears may be examined to monitor the progress of the cycle and to gauge the most appropriate time for mating – a procedure known as **exfoliative vaginal cytology**.

Vestibule – runs from the external urethral orifice to the outside at the **vulva**. It is shared by the reproductive and urinary tracts and so conducts both urine and fetuses to the outside. It has a similar structure to the vagina but the walls are not ridged by longitudinal folds.

Vulva – the external opening of the female tract. It consists of:
- the **labiae** – a pair of vertical lips joined dorsally and ventrally and forming a vertical slit known as the **vulval cleft**. Normally the lips are held together to prevent infection entering the tract, but in the bitch they become enlarged and relaxed during pro-oestrus and oestrus to allow mating. This does not occur in the queen.
- the **clitoris** – a knob-like structure of cavernous erectile tissue which lies just inside the ventral part of the vulval cleft.

MAMMARY GLANDS

These are modified cutaneous glands, which lie just under the skin on either side of the midline, on the ventral wall of the abdomen and thorax. The bitch has five pairs and the queen has four pairs. Mammary glands are also present in the male. Each gland consists of glandular tissue surrounded by connective tissue and lined by a secretory epithelium. Milk drains through a network of sinuses which eventually combine to form **teat canals**, each of which opens to the outside through a **teat orifice**. Each gland has one teat but each teat has several orifices.

The process of milk production is known as lactation and results from the interaction of three hormones:
- **Progesterone** – secreted by the corpus luteum in the ovary. Causes the mammary glands to enlarge during the early stages of pregnancy.
- **Prolactin** – secreted by the anterior pituitary gland (see Chapter 5) during the last third of pregnancy. Causes the glandular tissue to secrete milk, which remains within the teat sinuses.
- **Oxytocin** – secreted by the posterior pituitary gland (see Chapter 5) a few hours before and after parturition. When the neonate suckles or the teat is gently squeezed, a reflex arc initiates the secretion of oxytocin to cause the contraction of smooth muscle around the glands, and the milk is released or 'let down'.

MILK COMPOSITION

This varies with time and also depends on the species – the milk of the bitch and queen is more concentrated and contains more protein and twice as much fat as cow's milk. The milk that is secreted for about the first 48 hours after parturition is known as **colostrum** and is rich in maternal antibodies, which are proteins responsible for providing the neonate with immunity to diseases to which the dam has been exposed. It is vital that the neonate takes in the colostrum within the first 24 hours of life: during this time the antibodies are able to pass through the intestinal wall into the bloodstream unchanged. After this the antibodies are digested and destroyed. Maternal antibodies remain viable in the body for about 10–12 weeks, after which

Table 10.1 Average composition of milk

Constituent	Percentage content	Comments
Water	70–90	
Fat	0–30	Varies with species
Protein	1–15	Varies with species
Carbohydrate	3–7	Varies with species
Minerals	0.5–1	Calcium, phosphate, magnesium, sodium, potassium, chloride. Low in iron and copper. Traces of iodine, cobalt, tin and silica
Vitamins	Trace	A, B2, B5, E, K. Low in vitamins C and D

the young animal can produce antibodies of its own. Once the colostrum has stopped forming, the composition of milk becomes fairly constant (Table 10.1).

THE OESTROUS CYCLE

The oestrous cycle may be defined as the rhythmic phenomenon seen in all post-pubertal non-pregnant female animals, involving regular but limited periods of sexual receptivity known as oestrus.

The **functions** of the oestrous cycle are:
- To produce ova from the ovary ready to be fertilised by the spermatozoa of the male.
- To prepare the reproductive tract to receive the fertilised ova.
- To produce behavioural patterns in the female that advertise to the male that she is receptive.
- To cause the female to stand still and allow mating by the male.

Memory Jogger
You may notice as you read around the subject that the words associated with the oestrous cycle vary in their spelling. This is because 'oestrous' (pro-oestrous, metoestrous, anoestrous) is an adjective describing the cycle, while 'oestrus' (pro-oestrus, metoestrus, anoestrus) is a noun and is a phase of the cycle. In American textbooks 'oestrous' and 'oestrus' will be spelt 'estrous' and 'estrus'.

The oestrous cycle involves a series of simultaneous events within the ovary and the reproductive tract and in the female's behaviour patterns, all of which are linked by complicated hormonal pathways. The pattern and timing of the oestrous cycle vary between species – the cycle shown by the bitch is different from that shown by the queen.

The cycle is divided into several phases of different lengths:

- **Pro-oestrus** – preparation for oestrus, during which the developing ovarian follicles begin to secrete oestrogen.
- **Oestrus** – the period of sexual receptivity, during which the female will stand and allow herself to be mated.
- **Metoestrus** – the period during which the reproductive tract is under the influence of progesterone secreted by the corpus luteum within the ovary. May also be called dioestrus.
- **Anoestrus** – the period between oestrous cycles, during which there is little ovarian activity.

Memory Jogger

To remember the order in which the phases of the oestrous cycle occur, think of **POMA** – **p**ro-oestrus, **o**estrus, **m**etoestrus, **a**noestrus.

HORMONAL CONTROL OF THE OESTROUS CYCLE

The oestrous cycle is controlled by the complex interrelationship between several hormones produced by the pituitary gland and the ovary (Table 10.2).

The sequence of events is:

1. At the start of the breeding season or at puberty, external stimuli, such as light, environmental temperature or the presence of other animals, reach the brain through the ears, eyes and nose and affect the **hypothalamus** at the base of the brain. The hypothalamus secretes **gonadotrophin releasing hormone (GRH)** and the oestrous cycle begins.
2. GRH stimulates the **anterior pituitary gland** at the base of the forebrain to secrete **follicle stimulating hormone (FSH)**.
3. FSH acts on the **ovaries** and stimulates the primary follicles to become ripe **Graafian follicles**, each containing an ovum. The follicular tissue around the ovum secretes **oestrogen**.

Table 10.2 Hormones involved in the control of the oestrous cycle

Hormone	Action
Gonadotrophin releasing hormone (GRH)	Produced by the hypothalamus in the response to external stimuli. Stimulates the release of gonadotrophins from the pituitary gland
Follicle-stimulating hormone (FSH)	Produced by the anterior pituitary gland. Stimulates the development of follicles within the ovary
Luteinising hormone (LH) Gonadotrophin	Produced by the anterior pituitary gland. Acts on the mature follicles in the ovary, bringing about ovulation and the conversion of the remaining follicular tissue to a corpus luteum
Oestrogen	Produced by the mature follicles. Initiates the behavioural patterns seen during pro-oestrus and oestrus; prepares the reproductive tract for mating. Inhibits further secretion of FSH and stimulates secretion of LH
Progesterone	Produced by the mature follicle just before ovulation and by the corpus luteum. Prepares the reproductive tract to receive the fertilised ova; enlarges the mammary glands. Inhibits further production of GRH

4. Oestrogen produces the behaviour associated with pro-oestrus and prepares the reproductive tract for mating.

5. Oestrogen also inhibits further production of FSH by negative feedback (see Chapter 5), thus preventing any more follicles from maturing, and stimulates the secretion of **luteinising hormone (LH)**.

6. LH is secreted by the **anterior pituitary gland** and acts on the Graafian follicles, causing them to **ovulate**, i.e. to release the ova. It also luteinises or changes the remaining follicular tissue to form corpora lutea (singular **corpus luteum**), which secrete **progesterone**.

7. Falling levels of oestrogen and rising levels of progesterone produce the behavioural signs of oestrus and make the female stand still, allowing her to be mated.

8. Progesterone prepares the reproductive tract to receive the fertilised ova and causes enlargement of the mammary glands.

9. Progesterone also inhibits production of GRH by negative feedback; this prevents further oestrous cycles until the corpus luteum regresses and the whole cycle begins again.

OVULATION

This is the process by which an ovum or egg is released from its follicle within the ovary. At birth, the ovary of the female animal contains all the germ cells that she will ever use in her lifetime, and these act as a reservoir from which the follicles will develop at the onset of sexual maturity or **puberty**. In multiparous species such as the dog and cat, many follicles will develop in each ovary during each oestrous cycle. Each mature follicle, known as a **Graafian follicle**, consists of an outer double layer of cells surrounding a small amount of fluid and an **ovum** formed by the process of meiosis (see Chapter 1). These follicles secrete the hormone **oestrogen**. When the follicle has reached its full size, it ruptures or **ovulates** to release the ovum, which passes down the uterine tube. The remaining follicular tissue becomes luteinised to form the **corpus luteum**, which secretes the hormone **progesterone**.

OESTROUS CYCLE OF THE BITCH

- The bitch reaches **puberty** at about 6 months of age but there is variation depending on the breed – smaller breeds mature earlier than larger breeds. Puberty is marked by the first day of the first oestrous cycle.
- The bitch is described as being **monoestrous**, which means that during each period of ovarian activity there is one period of oestrus or sexual receptivity.
- The bitch commonly has one or two oestrous cycles per year, i.e. comes into 'season' or is 'on heat' every 6 months, but there is wide variation.
- There is no recognisable breeding season in the bitch.
- The bitch is a **spontaneous ovulator**, which means that she ovulates at the same point in each cycle regardless of whether or not she has been mated. The bitch ovulates on approximately the tenth day of the cycle.

During the cycle the bitch shows the following signs:

Pro-oestrus – lasts approximately nine days. The vulva becomes enlarged and there is a blood-stained vaginal discharge – some bitches lick this away so it may not always be seen. The presence of the discharge marks day 1 of the cycle.

The bitch is 'flirty' and excitable and is attractive to male dogs but she will not allow mating. She may urinate more frequently, which helps to distribute her smell, thus advertising that she is in season.

Oestrus – approximately nine days. The vulva may continue to swell and the discharge becomes straw-coloured. The excitable behaviour continues and the bitch may escape to find a dog. She will now allow mating to take place. Ovulation, which is not detectable externally, occurs during the first or second day of oestrus or the tenth day of the complete cycle.

Metoestrus – approximately 90 days, during which the tract is influenced by progesterone. In the bitch we can divide it into two phases:

- **Metoestrus I** – lasts for approximately 20 days. Begins when the bitch refuses mating and ends when all external signs have returned to normal. The discharge dries up, the vulva shrinks and the bitch's behaviour returns to normal.
- **Metoestrus II** – lasts for approximately 70 days. There are no external or behavioural signs but internally the corpus luteum remains in the ovary and continues to secrete progesterone. It is during this phase that a false pregnancy may occur.

Anoestrus – lasts approximately 3–9 months, but there is wide individual variation. During this phase the behaviour and appearance of the bitch are normal.

Towards the end of anoestrus, follicles begin to develop within the ovary and to secrete oestrogen. When the amount of oestrogen has risen to a significant level it will initiate the behavioural signs of pro-oestrus.

Table 10.3 provides a summary of all the events of the oestrous cycle of the bitch.

Memory Jogger

To help you make sense of the oestrous cycle and to help you correlate all the events that occur simultaneously, look at Table 10.3 for a summary.

Table 10.3 Summary of events that occur within the oestrous cycle of the bitch

Phases of the oestrous cycle	External and behavioural signs	Events in the ovary	Reproductive tract	Hormones
Pro-oestrus – approx. 9 days	Enlarged vulva, blood-stained vaginal discharge. Flirty, excitable behaviour. Will not allow mating	Follicles develop and mature into Graafian follicles	Vagina becomes thickened and moist ready for mating	Oestrogen secreted by the follicles
Oestrus – approx. 9 days	Enlarged vulva, straw-coloured vaginal discharge. Excitable, may try to escape and find a male. Will stand for mating	Mature follicles ovulate on 1st or 2nd day (10th day of cycle). Remaining follicular tissue becomes luteinised to form corpora lutea	Vagina remains moist and thickened. Towards the end of the phase the endometrium of the uterus begins to thicken	Oestrogen levels fall and progesterone levels secreted by the corpora lutea rise
Metoestrus I – approx. 20 days	Vulva shrinks, discharge dries up. Behaviour gradually returns to normal	Corpus luteum remains in the ovary for the entire phase	Endometrium of the uterus becomes thickened and glandular to receive the fertilised ova if present	Progesterone levels remain high
Metoestrus II – approx. 70 days	Appearance and behaviour are normal	Corpus luteum remains in the ovary for about 35 days (55 days in total)	Endometrium is thickened and glandular. Mammary glands may enlarge slightly. If bitch is not pregnant there is a gradual return to normal	Progesterone levels remain high until corpora lutea regress
Anoestrus – approx 3–9 months	Appearance and behaviour are normal	No activity. Just before the start of the next cycle, a few primary follicles will start to enlarge	Reproductive tract is normal	Levels of oestrogen and progesterone are very low, but towards the end of anoestrus, levels of FSH are detectable and oestrogen levels start to rise

If the bitch is pregnant, the corpus luteum remains in the ovary and secretes progesterone for about 55 days. If the animal is not pregnant, the corpus luteum remains for almost as long and the reproductive tract remains under the influence of progesterone. In some bitches this gives rise to the condition known as a **false pregnancy, pseudopregnancy or pseudocyesis**. The bitch thinks she is pregnant and starts to mother soft toys or slippers as if they were her puppies. She may become anorexic and may produce milk. Treatment includes hormone treatment or, if the condition recurs at every season, ovariohysterectomy may be recommended.

OESTROUS CYCLE OF THE QUEEN

- The queen reaches puberty at about 6 months of age, but this depends on the time of year in which the kitten was born. Most queens come into season in the early spring after they were born so a kitten born in late summer may only be 5 months old at puberty.
- The queen is described as being **seasonally polyoestrous** because she has many periods of oestrus or sexual receptivity within one breeding season.
- The **breeding season** of the cat is between January or February and September. However, many cats are kept in centrally heated houses, which may induce them to come into season at any time of the year.
- The queen is an **induced ovulator**, which means that she will only ovulate in response to the stimulus of mating. Ovulation occurs within about 36 hours after mating.

During the cycle the queen shows the following signs:

(There is no pro-oestrus phase in the queen.)

Oestrus – lasts for 4–7 days. There are no external physical signs but behavioural signs include **lordosis** – putting the rump in the air with the tail to one side, an increase in affectionate behaviour and **calling** – a loud yowling noise that advertises to tomcats far and wide that she is receptive.

Dioestrus – approximately 14 days. The queen's behaviour returns to normal. As the queen is an induced ovulator, if mating has not occurred there is no formation of a corpus luteum or progesterone secretion and the ovary is simply inactive for the short period of dioestrus. Follicles begin to develop and secrete oestrogen again just before oestrus starts.

Throughout the breeding season the queen will have alternate periods of oestrus and dioestrus until the non-breeding season occurs. The only event that will stop this is conception and pregnancy.

Anoestrus – approximately 4 months. The queen's behaviour is normal and the ovary remains inactive through the winter months. In early spring, follicles begin to develop and the queen goes into oestrus.

MULTIPLE CHOICE

Now use these multiple choice questions to test your under-standing of this chapter.

1. Spermatozoa are produced within the seminiferous tubules of the testis by:

a. mydriasis ○
b. mitosis ○
c. myiasis ○
d. meiosis. ○

2. Which of the following structures is seen in the reproductive system of the tomcat but NOT in that of the dog?

a. testes ○
b. prostate gland ○
c. bulbourethral glands ○
d. ductus deferens. ○

3. An animal that gives birth to several young at the same time is described as being:

a. multiparous ○
b. multigravid ○
c. precocial ○
d. bicornuate. ○

4. The part of the peritoneum that suspends the uterine tube within the abdominal cavity is the:

a. mesometrium ○

b. mesovarium ○

c. broad ligament ○

d. mesosalpinx. ○

5. Which of these statements best describes the reproductive pattern of the bitch?

a. The bitch is an induced ovulator and is monoestrous. ○

b. The bitch is a spontaneous ovulator and is monoestrous. ○

c. The bitch is an induced ovulator and is seasonally polyoestrous. ○

d. The bitch is a spontaneous ovulator and is seasonally polyoestrous. ○

6. Which hormones are involved in the process of lactation?

a. oestrogen and progesterone ○

b. FSH and oestrogen ○

c. prolactin and GRH ○

d. oxytocin and prolactin. ○

THE ANSWERS ARE:

1 d, 2 c, 3 a, 4 d, 5 b, 6 d.

11
The Integument

The integument is the largest organ in the body and forms its outer covering. Although it comprises such apparently different structures as hair, skin and claws, they are all based around a common tissue design. The principal function of the integument is protection, which is why there is such variation in the parts of the integument: where an area needs a greater degree of protection, the tissue is thick and hard – the claws, for example – but in areas that need less protection or are also protected by other structures, the tissue is much thinner and more delicate.

The **parts** of the integument are the:
- skin
- nosepad
- footpads
- claws
- hair.

The **functions** of the integument are:
- **Protection** – forms a barrier to protect the internal environment from the changing and sometimes hostile external environment. The different parts of the integument have various protective functions:
  - **Skin** – thicker in areas that are the most vulnerable to physical damage, such as around the scruff of the neck, which is often the site of dog bites. Provides an intact, impermeable barrier protecting against water and electrolyte loss and against the absorption of water and harmful toxins. Protects against invasion by harmful pathogens.
  - **Claws** – form a hard covering over the distal phalanx of each digit.
  - **Footpads** – form protective cushions that protect the weight-bearing surface of the foot.
  - **Hair** – gives added protection to the skin and grows more thickly in more vulnerable areas, such as the scruff of the neck.

- **Thermoregulation** – maintains the body temperature within a normal range by providing:
  - A good blood supply within the skin – vasodilatation of the capillaries conducts heat from the body's core to the surface, from which it is radiated away. Vasoconstriction conserves heat within the body.
  - A covering of erectile hairs – traps a layer of warm air close to the skin.
  - A layer of adipose tissue – fat cells within the hypodermis insulate the body against heat loss.
  - Sweat glands – secrete sweat, which evaporates and cools the skin surface.
- **Sensation** – the skin is able to monitor the external environment by means of sensory nerve endings that are sensitive to touch, pain and pressure. This information is then transmitted to the central nervous system, where it is interpreted and a response is made (see Chapter 4).
- **Storage** – adipose tissue within the hypodermis also acts as an energy store.
- **Secretion** – the skin contains many different types of exocrine glands, which secrete their products onto the surface:
  - **Sebum** – secreted by **sebaceous glands** onto the skin and hair, which keeps them supple and waterproofed. Modified sebaceous glands include anal sacs (see Chapter 8), ceruminous glands in the ear canal (see Chapter 4) and Meibomian glands around the eyelids (see Chapter 4).
  - **Sweat** – secreted by **sweat or sudoriferous glands** onto the surface of the skin; sweat evaporates and causes cooling.
  - **Milk** – secreted by the **mammary glands**, which are highly modified and enlarged sweat glands (see Chapter 10).
  - **Precursor of vitamin D** – secreted by the skin and, when acted upon by ultraviolet light from the sun, is converted into vitamin D. This is then activated by enzymes in the kidneys and liver and affects the uptake of calcium from the intestine.

- **Communication** – specialised glands around the anus and the head secrete pheromones or 'smelly hormones', which provide information about personal identity, territorial ownership and reproductive state to other members of the same species. Erectile hairs around the neck and along the spine are used by the dog to threaten or warn other dogs, while cats fluff up their tails as a warning of their aggressive mood.

STRUCTURE OF THE INTEGUMENT

The structure of the **skin** shows the fundamental pattern on which the structure of all other parts of the integument is based. The skin (Fig. 11.1) consists of three layers:

- epidermis
- dermis
- hypodermis.

EPIDERMIS

This is the outermost layer of stratified squamous epithelium. Can be divided into:

- **Stratum germinativum** – the basal layer, lying closest to the dermis. The cells divide by **mitosis** (see Chapter 1) to form new cells, which are then pushed upwards by more cells forming beneath them.
- **Stratum granulosum** – the middle layer. The cells become more oval, lose their organelles and eventually die. They develop increasing amounts of the protective protein **keratin**, which

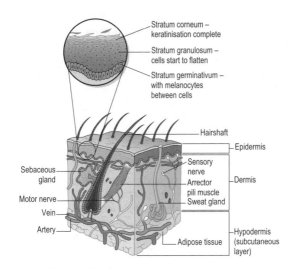

Figure 11.1 Structure of the skin

makes the skin tougher and more able to withstand chemical and physical damage. In pigmented skin, cells containing the dark pigment **melanin** are found in this layer.

● **Stratum corneum** – the top layer. The cells are flattened, enucleated and keratinised or cornified, creating a tough protective surface for the body. These cells or **squames** eventually slough off.

The epidermis varies in thickness depending on the area of the body and the degree of protection required. The epidermis of the footpad is many cells thick to protect the weight-bearing surface of the foot, while the areas of skin covered with hair may consist of only three or four layers of cells. Here there is very little wear and a covering of hair provides additional protection. In some parts of the integument the lower layers of the epidermis project into the dermis forming **dermal papillae**. These prevent the epidermis tearing away from the dermis when it takes weight or is subjected to friction.

DERMIS

Also called the **corium**, this layer attaches the epidermis to the underlying tissues. (Fig. 11.1). It is composed of irregular, dense fibrous connective tissue (see Chapter 2) containing a variety of cells, including **fibroblasts, collagen fibres** to give strength, **elastic fibres** to provide stretch, **hair follicles, blood capillaries** and **nerve fibres. Sebaceous glands** secrete sebum directly into the hair follicles and simple coiled **sweat glands** open onto the surface of the skin and into the hair follicles. In the dog and the cat the only truly active sweat glands are found on the footpads and on the nosepad, so panting is the most important means of heat regulation.

HYPODERMIS

This layer, also called the **subcutaneous layer**, blends with the dermis. It consists of areolar or loose connective tissue (see Chapter 2), which allows the muscle and bone of the body to move freely without pulling on the overlying skin. The tissue has a good supply of blood capillaries and nerve fibres, and it is here that a layer of adipose tissue acts as an energy supply and as an insulating layer.

Memory Jogger

Modified cutaneous or skin glands include anal glands, mammary glands, sweat glands, sebaceous glands, ceruminous glands and Meibomian glands.

Modified epidermal structures include hair, claws, footpads and, in other species, horn and hooves.

MODIFIED EPIDERMAL STRUCTURES

Some areas of the skin are totally hairless and these are modified to provide extra protection.

NOSEPAD

Also called the **rhinarium**, this protects the bony end of the nasal chambers. It consists of a pad of thickened keratinised epidermis that is usually pigmented and well supplied with numerous glands, giving the nose its wet look.

FOOTPADS

These cover the joints within the distal extremities and thus protect the weight-bearing surfaces. Each pad consists of a thickened, keratinised and pigmented **epidermal pad** with deep dermal papillae. In the dog, the surface is roughened by conical papillae which provide grip during locomotion; in the cat the surface is smoother. Beneath the pad is a layer of dermal and adipose tissue which absorbs the force of concussion. Active sweat glands open onto the surface of the pad. There are seven pads on each fore foot and five on each hind foot:

- **Carpal or stop pad** – just distal to the carpal bones. Only on the fore foot.
- **Digital pads** – one pad overlying each distal interphalangeal joint, including the joint of the dew claw on the fore foot.
- **Metacarpal/metatarsal pads** – protect the phalangeal–metacarpal and phalangeal–metatarsal joints. In the dog the pad is heart-shaped and in the cat it is round.

CLAWS

These cover and extend beyond the **ungual process** of the distal phalanx of each digit. Their function is to protect the underlying bone and to provide grip during locomotion. In the cat they are also used as weapons of offence. The cells of the epidermis are often pigmented and contain a high proportion of keratin, creating a hard material called **horn**, which is resistant to physical and chemical damage.

Each claw is a laterally flattened beak-shaped structure. The two lateral surfaces form the **walls** of the claw, which enclose on the ventral surface a softer area of horn known as the **sole**. The claw grows from the **coronary border**, which rests under the **ungual crest** of each distal phalanx and is a specialised area of epidermis fitting into a groove of hairless epidermis known as the **claw fold**. The periosteum of the distal phalanx is continuous with the dermis of the claw, and together they fill the space between the outer epidermis and the ungual process. The dermis is vascular and forms the 'quick' of the claw.

The claws of the cat are sharper than those of the dog and are usually unpigmented. At rest they are retracted into the claw fold, which is achieved by the action of an **elastic ligament** running from the middle to the distal phalanx of each digit.

HAIR

Most of the body of the dog and cat has a thick covering of

hair but some areas, such as the scrotum, the ventral abdomen and the teats, have a relatively sparse covering. Some breeds of dog, such as the Mexican Hairless and the Chinese Crested, and the cat known as the Sphinx are almost totally hairless, which has been achieved by years of selective breeding.

Hair formation

Each hair is a modified epidermal structure growing from an individual hair **follicle**, formed from epidermal cells that dip down into the dermis. At the base of the follicle is the **bulb**, within which a knot of blood capillaries or the **dermal papilla** provides nutrients to the growing hair cells. The cells within the bulb divide to produce the keratinised hair **shaft**, which grows up through the centre of the follicle until it penetrates the skin surface. As each hair becomes old and falls out, a replacement hair develops from a new follicle.

Opening into each hair follicle is a **sebaceous gland**, which coats the hair with sebum to keep it supple and waterproof. Close to the base of each follicle is a band of smooth muscle known as the **arrector pili muscle**. As it contracts it pulls the hair upright. This process of **piloerection** traps a layer of warm air close to the skin. It is also used to raise the hackles of a dog or fluff up the tail of a cat to threaten or warn other animals.

Hair types

There are three main types:

- **Guard hairs** – form the outer layer of the coat. They are thicker, longer and stiffer than the hairs of the undercoat and are found over most of the body in broad tracts that follow the body contours and create a smooth appearance. Their function is to prevent water penetrating to the undercoat by causing it to run off; this is a particular feature of the coats of gundogs.

- **Wool hairs** – lie close to the body surface, creating the undercoat. They are thinner, softer and wavier than the guard hairs and their function is to warm and insulate the body. Breeds that are able to survive in subnormal temperatures, such as the Husky, have a dense overcoat and undercoat, while breeds such as the Doberman have almost no undercoat at all.

- **Sinus or tactile hairs** – include the vibrissae or 'whiskers'.

They are longer and coarser than other types of hair and are found mainly on the head associated with the sense organs. They are the first hairs formed in the embryo. At the base of each hair is a blood-filled sinus with a good supply of nerve fibres, which intensify any movement of the hair and convey the information to the central nervous system.

Hair growth

The neonate is born with a full coat of single hairs produced from primary follicles. As the animal matures, secondary hairs develop from the same follicles arranged in a crescent around each primary hair. This continues until puberty, by which time there may be six to ten hairs arising from one follicle. This 'puppy or kitten coat' is later replaced by the coarser adult coat.

Hair growth occurs in an annual cycle and is followed by **moulting** or **shedding**. Hair growth is affected by seasonal factors, such as temperature and photoperiod and the coat type changes – in summer the coat is thinner and more shiny or medullated, whereas in winter it is thicker and woollier. Moulting normally occurs twice a year, in spring and autumn, but because many animals are kept in centrally heated houses moulting may begin at any time of the year. Hair growth and quality are also affected by hormones, nutrition and general health.

MULTIPLE CHOICE

Now use these multiple choice questions to test your understanding of this chapter:

1. Which of the following plays a part in thermoregulation?

a. sebaceous glands ○
b. claws ○
c. hair ○
d. Meibomian glands. ○

2. The digital pads in the dog and cat are designed to protect the:

a. hock joint ○
b. distal interphalangeal joint ○
c. carpal joint ○
d. phalangeal–metacarpal joint. ○

3. Which of the following are modified cutaneous glands?

a. mammary and anal glands ○
b. adrenal and gastric glands ○
c. meibomian and pituitary glands ○
d. sweat and thyroid glands. ○

4. In which layer of the skin would you expect to find evidence of mitosis?

a. dermis ○
b. stratum corneum ○
c. hypodermis ○
d. stratum germinativum. ○

5. Which vitamin is formed within the skin?

a. vitamin A ○
b. vitamin B ○
c. vitamin C ○
d. vitamin D. ○

6. In the embryo which of the following hairs are formed first?

a. guard hairs ○
b. wool hairs ○
c. sinus hairs ○
d. down hairs. ○

THE ANSWERS ARE:

1 c, 2 b, 3 a, 4 d, 5 d, 6 c.

12

Comparative Anatomy – Birds, Reptiles and Fish

Nowadays many people keep exotic species as pets and for the welfare and treatment of these animals it is important to understand their anatomy and physiology. Let's use what you have learnt in the previous chapters about the dog and cat to study and compare the anatomy and physiology of some very different species.

THE BIRD

Birds all belong to the class Aves, which comprises about 8500 species. The common feature of members of this class is that they have an outer covering of feathers. Most birds are able to fly, exceptions being species such as the penguin, the kiwi and the ill-fated dodo. Much of the anatomy and physiology of birds shows adaptations to life in the air.

Memory Jogger
Look back to Chapter 1 and revise how all living organisms are classified by the binomial system invented by Carl Linnaeus.

FEATHERS

Feathers derive from epidermal cells in a similar way to the hairs of mammals. They are made of keratin and provide a strong but lightweight covering over the body and the wing.

Each feather consists of a central **shaft** or **rachis**, which gives off a series of branches or **barbs**. These in turn give off **barbules**, which interlock to form a flattened, wind-resistant surface. The feathers must be kept in optimum condition to function effectively, so birds constantly 'zip' up the barbules and apply oil from the preen gland at the base of the tail to keep them waterproof.

There are **four types** of feather:
- **Flight feathers** (primary and secondary) – long and rigid,

attached to the wing and tail. **Primary** feathers attach to digit 3 and to the fused metacarpals and provide the main thrust during flight. **Secondaries** are shorter than the primaries and are attached to the ulna.

- **Contour feathers** – cover the remainder of the wing and the outermost layer of the body producing a smooth outline. They are shorter and more flexible; the lower part of the vane is fluffy.
- **Down and filoplume** – lie under the contour feathers close to the body, creating an insulating layer. They are fluffy in appearance as they have no barbs. Filoplume are designed to break up, creating dust that absorbs sweat and dirt.

Adult birds **moult** annually, usually just after the breeding season. Moulting occurs over a period, and during this time the ability to fly may be impaired. This makes the bird vulnerable to predators.

Memory Jogger

Go back to Chapter 3 and compare the skeleton of the dog with the skeleton of the bird shown in Fig. 12.1. They are very obviously different, but both show adaptations to their own particular lifestyle.

MUSCULOSKELETAL SYSTEM

The skeleton of the bird (Fig. 12.1) is unlike that of any other animal. Many of its characteristic features are designed to reduce the weight of the skeleton while retaining the strength required for powered flight. The following points are significant.

- The weight of individual bones is reduced by having a **thinner cortex**, and many bones are hollow. To provide extra strength, the interior of the larger bones is reinforced by bony **struts** running across the central cavity.
- Some of the larger bones are **pneumatic** and are filled with air sacs that connect to the respiratory system.
- The sternum is laterally flattened to form the **keel**, which provides a large surface for the attachment of flight muscles.
- The number of **joints** in the body is reduced.
- The neck is long and mobile and contains more **cervical vertebrae** than the standard seven that are seen in all mammals.

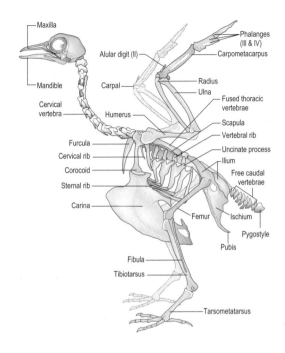

Figure 12.1 Skeleton of the pigeon

- The number of **coccygeal or caudal vertebrae** is reduced and they are fused to form the tail or **pygostyle**, to which the tail feathers are attached. At the base is the **preen gland** or **uropygial gland**.
- There is a single body cavity – birds have **no diaphragm**.
- There is no **floor** to the pelvic cavity, which enables the caudal part of the pelvis to hinge open and release the eggs.
- Birds do not have teeth, which have been replaced by a lightweight **beak** that is adapted to the eating habits of different species.
- In the skull the **orbit**, which houses the large eye, is large

and thin-walled and connects with large optic lobes in the brain.

- The forelimb is modified to form the **wing**. The bones are reduced to a humerus, separate ulna and radius, fused carpal and metacarpal bones and two digits. **Digit 3** is the main digit and carries the primary feathers, while **digit 1** carries a few feathers and is known as the **alula or bastard wing**.
- The **leg** contains some fused bones that form a tibiotarsus and a tarsometatarsus.
- Most birds have three forward-pointing **toes** and one toe that points backwards, but members of the parrot family have two toes forwards and two pointing backwards.

CARDIOVASCULAR SYSTEM

The cardiovascular system follows a similar plan to that of the mammal. The **four-chambered heart** lies within the cranial part of the body cavity. Birds have a **renal portal system** by which blood from the caudal end of the body can be diverted either directly into the caudal vena cava and so to the heart or to the kidneys, in a similar pattern to that of reptiles. There is a large blood supply to the flight muscles via the pectoral and brachial arteries. Within the blood, the **erythrocytes** or red blood corpuscles are oval and nucleated. Sites of venepuncture are shown in Table 12.1 (see p.191).

RESPIRATORY SYSTEM

The respiratory system of the bird (Fig. 12.2) is very different from that of the mammal and is adapted to meet the physiological needs of the bird when it is flying at speed or at high altitude, where oxygen levels are low.

The passage of air is as follows:
1. Air is drawn into the body by the movement of the muscles that form the body wall. There is **no diaphragm** in the bird.
2. It enters the body via a pair of external **nostrils or nares** or through the mouth. Some species have a cleft in the hard palate known as the **choana**, which connects the oral and nasal cavities. The nasal cavities contain **conchae**, which warm and moisten the inspired air.

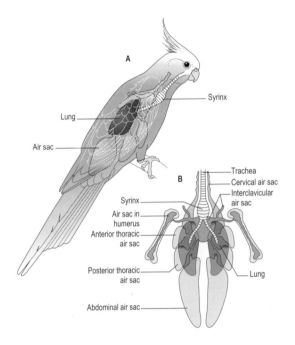

Labels on image A: Syrinx, Lung, Air sac

Labels on image B: Trachea, Cervical air sac, Interclavicular air sac, Syrinx, Air sac in humerus, Anterior thoracic air sac, Posterior thoracic air sac, Abdominal air sac, Lung

Figure 12.2 Respiratory system of the bird

3. Air passes down the **glottis**, which lies on the floor of the oral cavity, then travels through the complex **larynx** and down the **trachea** to its bifurcation into the **right and left bronchi**. At this point the trachea dilates to form a structure known as the **syrinx**, which plays a part in the production of sound.

4. Air passes into the relatively dense **lungs**, which are closely applied to the dorsal body wall. During respiration they do not expand in the same way as the lungs of mammals.

5. Within the lung tissue, each primary bronchus divides into smaller and smaller bronchi and into cylindrical parallel tubes known as **parabronchi**. Air capillaries surrounded by pulmonary capillaries penetrate through the walls of the parabronchi, and it is here that gaseous exchange takes place.

6. Air continues through the lungs and passes into thin-walled air sacs. Most species have nine **air sacs**, which occupy space within the body cavity and are also found within the larger bones. They act as a reservoir of air and act like bellows, pushing air back through the lungs. They also lighten the skeleton, so aiding flight.

7. Air returns from the air sacs and passes through the lungs for a second time. It is on this second passage that most gaseous exchange takes place.

DIGESTIVE SYSTEM

Within the class Aves, the specific anatomy of the digestive tract depends on the type of diet. This may be carnivorous, herbivorous, omnivorous, granivorous or fructivorous, but the basic pattern of the tract remains more or less the same. Food enters the tract via the oral cavity and passes down the tract as follows:

1. **Oral cavity** – food is picked up and broken into small pieces by the beak and the **tongue**. The shape of the **beak** is suited to the type of food eaten by the particular species. Within the oral cavity food is mixed with saliva from the **salivary glands**, but birds are unable to chew their food. **Taste buds** are located at the back of the oral cavity.

2. **Oesophagus and crop** – food passes down the thin-walled, distensible **oesophagus**, which lies on the right side of the neck and leads to the **crop**. The crop is a diverticulum of the oesophagus and lies outside the body cavity. It acts mainly as a storage organ but in some species, such as doves and pigeons, the epithelial lining secretes 'crop milk' to feed the young in the first few days of life.

3. **Stomach** – this consists of two parts:
   • **Proventriculus** – here food is stored and mixed with digestive juices secreted by gastric glands lining the walls.
   • **Gizzard** – a thick-walled muscular organ that grinds and mixes the food with digestive enzymes and grit or small stones taken in as part of the diet. The resulting mixture is physically broken down and partially digested.

4. **Small intestine** – food leaves the gizzard by the pylorus and enters the **duodenum** and **ileum**. The **pancreas** lies

in the duodenal loop. Birds have a relatively large, bilobed **liver** and some species have a **gall bladder**.

5. **Large intestine** – consists of a pair of blind-ending **caeca** (singular caecum) at the junction of the small and large intestine, a **rectum** and a **cloaca**. Bacterial digestion occurs within the caeca. The caeca are large and important in herbivorous and granivorous species but rudimentary in carnivorous species. The rectum is short and terminates at the cloaca. This is a common exit for the digestive, reproductive and urinary tracts.

REPRODUCTIVE SYSTEM

- **Female tract** (Fig. 12.3) – the tract comprises a pair of **ovaries** and **oviducts** leading to the **cloaca**. In many species the left ovary and oviduct are functional while the right side is vestigial. During the breeding season, ova, each consisting of an oocyte surrounded by a yolk, are released from the ovary and pass down the oviduct; one ovum is released approximately every 24 hours. The oviduct is divided into different regions, each of which makes a contribution to the finished egg:

  - **Infundibulum** – the funnel-shaped end of the oviduct; it collects the ovum from the ovary. Here fertilisation takes place and the first layer of albumen is added.

  - **Magnum** – the walls are glandular and the lumen is large. Most of the albumen is added here.

  - **Isthmus** – the walls consist of thick layers of circular muscle. Inner and outer shell membranes are added.

  - **Shell gland or uterus** – the walls contain longitudinal muscle and are lined with goblet cells. The shell undergoes calcification over a period of about 15 hours.

The finished egg passes through a sphincter muscle known as the **vagina** and is laid via the **cloaca**.

- **Male tract** – consists of a pair of **testes**, each of which is connected to the **cloaca** by a **vas deferens**. The testes of the bird are internal and are attached to the body wall cranial to the kidneys. **Spermatogenesis** occurs within the seminiferous tubules of the testes. Mature sperm pass down the vas deferens and out of the body via a modi-

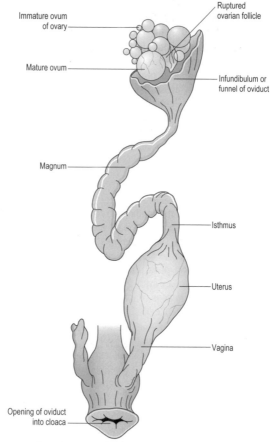

Figure 12.3 Reproductive tract of the female bird

fied area in the wall of the cloaca known as the **phallus**. The size of the phallus or rudimentary penis varies with the species of bird.

Sexual differentiation

The method of determining the sex of a bird depends on the species. The following methods may be used:

- **Sexual dimorphism** – the two sexes differ in external appearance; e.g. male and female mallards, and male and female pheasants. Only seen in some species of bird.

- **DNA testing** – examination of the chromosomes using a blood sample or cells taken from a growing feather.
- **Surgical sexing** – endoscopic examination of the internal gonads.

REPTILES

There are approximately 6500 species of reptiles, all of which are cold-blooded, covered in some form of scaly skin, and breed on land. They are divided into four orders but only two include species kept as exotic pets. These are:

1. **Order Chelonia** – the shelled reptiles (referred to as chelonians), such as tortoises, terrapins and turtles. (In the USA all shelled reptiles are described as turtles.)
2. **Order Squamata** – includes the **suborder Sauria** (lizards) and the **suborder Serpentes** (snakes).

All these species have a shared evolutionary route and therefore have many anatomical and physiological features in common. Within each body system we will look at the general anatomy and then look at the specific adaptations.

INTEGUMENT

The skin of reptiles is keratinised and thick and may be protected by scales. Reptiles grow by shedding or sloughing their skin – a process known as **ecdysis**. Underneath the old skin is a new layer that is soft at first; this allows rapid growth but leaves the reptile vulnerable to attack or damage until the layer hardens. Changes in the normal pattern of shedding may be an indicator of disease.

- **Chelonians** – characterised by a hard outer **shell** made up of keratinised plates or **scutes**. These plates are named according to the area they cover and each one grows annually by adding a ring to the outside, so that the overall size of the shell increases. The markings on the shell of each individual animal are different and can be used as a means of identification. The upper component of the shell or **carapace** is domed and the ventral component or **plastron** is flattened. Together they form a box-like structure that protects the internal organs.
- **Lizards** – covered in thick scaly skin that forms a smooth outline. In many species the skin is shed in pieces and

some species of lizard, such as geckos, will eat the sloughed skin. Some lizards, notably the chameleons, are able to change their skin colour to camouflage themselves. The gecko family is characterised by having fine overlapping scales or **lamellae** on the soles of their feet, which enable them to walk over apparently smooth surfaces, such as glass.

- **Snakes** – the scales vary according to the region of the body. Those on the dorsal and lateral parts of the body are small while those on the more ventral parts are larger and thicker. Snakes do not have movable eyelids like those of mammals, but instead the upper and lower eyelids are fused to form a transparent **spectacle** over the cornea. During ecdysis the skin becomes dull and an early indication of shedding may be that the spectacle becomes cloudy. The skin over the spectacles lifts off, the skin over the head splits and the snake crawls out of the entire outer layer of old skin.

SKELETAL SYSTEM

Reptiles are vertebrates and have an internal skeleton that bears some resemblance to that of the mammals.

- **Chelonians** – the pectoral and pelvic girdles are enclosed within the shell and are directed vertically to provide support. There are ten vertebrae, which form the undersurface of the carapace.

- **Lizards** – the skeleton follows the basic plan seen in mammals but there is no sternum. Many species are able to show **autotomy** or the ability to shed the tail as a means of defence. The shed tail carries on wriggling, which diverts the attention of the predator while the lizard escapes. A new tail may grow to replace it but the new caudal vertebrae are cartilaginous rather than bony and the tail often regrows with a different colour.

- **Snakes** (Fig. 12.4) – these are legless and have an elongated body. The **skull** is complex and the mandibles of the lower jaw are able to separate widely, enabling the snake to ingest large items of prey. There are between 150 and 400 **vertebrae**, all with a similar shape and each one giving off a pair of **ribs**. These are fused to the vertebrae but are not joined in the ventral midline. Some species show evidence of vestigial limbs in the area of the pelvic girdle.

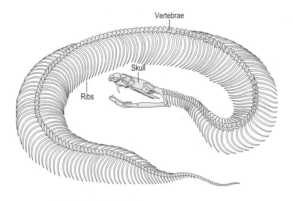

Figure 12.4 Skeleton of a typical snake

Externally these may be seen as spurs on either side of the vent.

CARDIOVASCULAR SYSTEM

The reptilian heart has **three chambers** – a right and a left atrium but only one ventricle. The ventricle is functionally but not anatomically divided into three subchambers and receives blood from both the right and the left atrium. Within the blood the **erythrocytes** or red blood corpuscles are nucleated in a similar way to those of the bird.

In the peripheral circulation reptiles have a **renal portal system**, which carries blood from the hind limbs and tail directly to the kidneys. This has clinical significance because any drug injected into the hind limbs or the tail may be excreted via the kidneys without reaching the remainder of the body (Table 12.1, see p. 191).

- **Chelonians** – auscultation of the heart may be difficult as the shell muffles the heart sounds. Sites for venepuncture include the jugular veins and the dorsal venous sinus in the dorsal midline of the tail.
- **Lizards** – have a large ventral abdominal vein. Sites for venepuncture include the cephalic vein in larger species and the ventral tail vein, but this should be avoided in species that show autotomy.
- **Snakes** – the heart is located at approximately one-third

of the length of the body. The site for venepuncture is the ventral venous sinus in the midline of the ventral tail.

Memory Jogger

Go back to Chapter 6 and compare the structure of the mammalian heart and circulation with that of the reptiles.

RESPIRATORY SYSTEM

Reptiles are able to extract oxygen from the air and the process of gaseous exchange is similar to that of mammals. Like birds, reptiles do not possess a **diaphragm**.

- **Chelonians** – the rigid shell prevents the body wall from expanding during respiration. Respiration is accomplished with the help of limb and head movements, which change the internal pressure in the body cavity. Air enters the body through a pair of **nostrils**. The **glottis** lies at the base of the tongue and the **trachea** is short, enabling the animal to breathe with its head retracted. The **lungs** lie dorsally in the body cavity; this provides buoyancy in aquatic species.
- **Lizards** – respiration is achieved by expansion and contraction of the ribs.
- **Snakes** – the **left lung** is either reduced in size or completely absent. The anterior part of the right lung is involved in gaseous exchange while the posterior part is avascular and forms an air sac that acts as a reserve during periods of apnoea.

DIGESTIVE SYSTEM

There is great variation in the digestive systems of reptiles but in all species the tract terminates at a **cloaca**. This is divided into three parts – the **coprodeum**, which collects faeces, the **urodeum**, which collects urinary waste, and the **proctodeum**, which is the final collecting chamber before the waste is eliminated. Lizards and snakes possess a structure in the roof of the mouth known as **Jacobson's organ**. The tongue is used to 'taste' the environment and is then brought into contact with the organ, which conveys the information via a branch of the olfactory nerve to the brain.

- **Chelonians** – teeth are replaced by a horny **beak**. The **tongue** is large and fleshy. The **oesophagus** runs down the left side of the neck and enters the **stomach**, which lies

Table 12.1 Sites for the administration of parenteral medicines in some exotic species

Type of injection	Birds	Chelonians	Lizards	Snakes
Intravenous	Brachial vein Jugular vein Medial metatarsal vein	Jugular vein Dorsal venous sinus	Cephalic vein Ventral tail vein	Ventral venous sinus
Intramuscular	Pectoral muscles	Triceps muscle in forelimb Pectoral muscles Hind limb muscles	Caudal muscles of the fore-limb Into the tail – watch out for autotomy!	Intercostal muscles
Subcutaneous	Under the skin over the breast	Under the loose skin of the neck	Under the loose skin over the ribs	Under the loose skin over the ribs

transversely across the body cavity. The **intestine** is relatively short and exits via the **cloaca**.

- **Lizards** – most lizards have **teeth** but they are attached to the side of the mandibles rather than lying in sockets. They are regularly shed and replaced. The **tongue** is used in conjunction with **Jacobson's organ** in the roof of the mouth. The anatomy of the digestive tract depends on the type of diet, which may be carnivorous, insectivorous, herbivorous or omnivorous. The simple **stomach** is elongated and a **caecum** is present in herbivorous species.

- **Snakes** – all species are carnivorous and have six pairs of undifferentiated **teeth** that are replaced regularly. Some species have **fangs** that are used to convey **venom** from specialised glands above the oral cavity into the prey. The **tongue** is thin and forked and is used in conjunction with **Jacobson's organ**. So that it can fit into the long body, the **stomach** is elongated. The **intestine** is relatively short, reflecting the carnivorous diet.

URINOGENITAL SYSTEM

Reptiles have a pair of kidneys without loops of Henle, which means that they are unable to concentrate their urine. Lizards and chelonians possess a thin-walled bladder in which the urine may change.

Chelonians – the urine produced is relatively unconcentrated. Males have a single large penis which protrudes from the cloaca.

- **Sexual differentiation**
  - Sexual dimorphism – visible differences in the external features.
  - Males have longer tails than females.
  - The plastron of the male is concave, while that of the female is flatter.
  - The caudal scute of the female is curved upwards.
  - The male terrapin has long front claws.

Lizards – males have paired copulatory organs or **hemipenes**, each of which is a closed hollow tube which lies folded up and inverted within the tail caudal to the cloaca. Only one hemipenis is used during copulation, when it is erected by blood and inserted into the cloaca of the female. Female lizards lay eggs, which are produced via the cloaca. There is no uterus.

- **Sexual differentiation**
  - Sexual dimorphism – depends on the species.
  - Males have a more swollen base of the tail to enclose the hemipenes.
  - Presence of femoral or pre-anal pores – pattern depends on species.

Snakes – there is no bladder and the ureters empty directly into the **urodeum** of the cloaca. Males have **hemipenes**, which lie invaginated within the base of the tail just caudal to the vent. Some species of snake are very slim and females of these species have only one **ovary** and **oviduct**. Snakes may be **oviparous**, meaning that they lay eggs, or are **viviparous,** i.e. they give birth to live young, which develop in the egg retained within the body.

- **Sexual differentiation**
  - Sexual dimorphism is seen in some species.
  - The tail, which is measured from the vent to the tip of the tail, is longer in the male than in the female.

- The area around the vent is more swollen in the male than in the female as it houses the hemipenes.
- Females are usually larger than males.
- Use of a probe – a well-lubricated rod is carefully inserted under the vent and directed towards the tail. In the male the probe will be able to pass down a longer distance than in the female.

Memory Jogger

Remember the characteristics of all chelonians:
· ectothermic or cold-blooded
· have four legs
· body is protected by a hard outer shell
· have a horny beak
· have eyelids and external eardrums
· oviparous
· may be terrestrial or aquatic
· aquatic species may live in fresh water (terrapins) or salt water (turtles).

Memory Jogger

Remember the characteristics of all lizards:
· ectothermic or cold-blooded
· have four legs
· have external eardrums
· have eyelids
· tongue 'tastes' the environment in conjunction with Jacobson's organ
· grow by shedding their skin – known as ecdysis
· some species show autotomy.

Memory Jogger

Remember the characteristics of all snakes:
· ectothermic or cold-blooded
· legless
· eyelids are fused and transparent to form a spectacle
· have no external eardrums or ears
· oviparous or viviparous
· can dislocate their upper and lower jaws
· tongue 'tastes' the environment in conjunction with Jacobson's organ
· grow by shedding their skin – known as ecdysis.

FISH

Fish are cold-blooded vertebrates that are adapted to live and breathe in water. There are over 30 000 species of fish, divided into the jawed and jawless fish. The jawed fish are further divided into the cartilaginous fish, such as the sharks and rays, and the bony fish, which include all types of ornamental aquarium fish. The bony fish include groups known as the higher and lower teleosts; despite being found in a range of habitats all over the world, they have a similar anatomy.

INTEGUMENT

Fish have a covering of overlapping flexible bony plates known as **scales**. These are covered with a layer of mucus that forms the **glycocalyx**, which helps movement through the water by reducing friction and also has a bactericidal and fungicidal action to protect against skin infections.

MUSCULOSKELETAL SYSTEM

The characteristic shape of the fish makes it streamlined for swimming through water. Movement is brought about by blocks of muscle or **myomeres** arranged on either side of the axial skeleton (Fig. 12.5). Their contractions bend the body laterally and generate the force to move forward. The bones of the **cranium** are rigid. The number of **vertebrae** varies; those in the thoracic region articulate with the ribs and support the lateral walls of the body cavity.

Locomotion is brought about by the use of **fins**, each of which consists of tissue stretched over rays. The rays may be stiff and unjointed or soft with many articulations. The shape of the fins, particularly that of the tail or caudal fin, provides an indication of the swimming habits of the species.

Buoyancy in the water is brought about by means of a gas-filled **swim bladder**, which lies within the body cavity just ventral to the vertebral column. The structure of the swim bladder depends on the species. That of the lower teleosts, such as the carp, salmon and catfish, is linked to the foregut and is refilled by the fish rising to the surface and taking a mouthful of air – this is a **physostomous** swim bladder. The swim bladder of the higher teleosts,

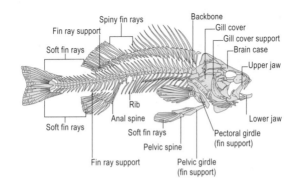

Figure 12.5 Skeleton of a fish

such as the perch and stickleback, becomes filled with carbon dioxide during larval development and remains present throughout the fish's life – this is a **physoclistous** swim bladder.

RESPIRATORY SYSTEM

This system is obviously very different from that of all the other species covered by this book as fish live in water. The ability to extract oxygen from the surrounding water is achieved by the presence of gills. There are five lateral **gill slits** on each side of the pharyngeal wall. Each gill consists of a bony **gill arch**, which supports vascularised **gill filaments**. These in turn give off **lamellae** or secondary filaments. On the pharyngeal side of each gill arch are elongated projections known as **gill rakers**, which protect the delicate gills from food particles that could cause damage. Externally the gills are protected by flaps known as **opercula** (singular operculum). Water is taken in through the mouth, passes over the gills, where gaseous exchange takes place, and is forced out through the opercula.

Nitrogenous waste is excreted in the form of **ammonia**, which is extremely toxic and is excreted only by organisms that live in a watery environment, which then dilutes it. The gills are the most important site of nitrogenous excretion; in this respect fish differ from mammals, which excrete nitrogenous waste in the form of urea from the kidneys.

CIRCULATORY SYSTEM

The circulation of the fish is described as being **single** because blood passes through the heart once in a complete circuit of the body (see Chapter 6). The **heart** consists of a single atrium and a ventricle, and is long and folded. Blood leaves the ventricle in the arterial system and is pumped to the gills; here it picks up oxygen, which is then conveyed to the tissues. On the return journey carbon dioxide is carried by the venous circulation to the gills, from where it is excreted. Blood then flows into the atrium of the heart.

Memory Jogger

Go back to Chapter 6 and look at the circulatory system of the mammal. Blood passes through the mammalian heart twice during a complete circuit of the body. This type of circulation is described as being double.

DIGESTIVE SYSTEM

The anatomy of the digestive tract depends on the diet of the species. Food is ingested by protrusion of the jaws, which creates a sucking movement. In addition, some predatory fish also have **teeth** which are used for catching and holding their prey. Food passes into a tube-like **stomach** and then into the **intestine**, which is a simple, short tube. Waste materials are excreted via the **rectum and anus**.

URINARY SYSTEM

The **kidneys** lie ventral to the spine and in some species may sit like a saddle on the swim bladder. They have many functions, including excretion, haemopoiesis, the secretion of hormones and osmoregulation.

REPRODUCTIVE SYSTEM

Most teleosts have **separate sexes** and there is wide variation in their reproductive patterns, which include hermaphroditism and parthenogenesis. Fertilisation may be **internal** or **external** depending on the species. Females may lay eggs (**oviparous**) or produce live young (**viviparous**).

MULTIPLE CHOICE

Now use these multiple choice questions to test your understanding of this chapter:

1. Which feathers attach to the ulna in the wing of a bird?

a. contour ○
b. filoplume ○
c. primaries ○
d. secondaries. ○

2. The toes of most birds are arranged:

a. three forward, two back ○
b. three forward, one back ○
c. one forward, three back ○
d. two forward, two back. ○

3. With reference to the respiratory tract of the bird, which statement is FALSE?

a. There is no diaphragm separating the thorax from the abdomen. ○
b. The lungs are flexible and spongy and lie close to the ventral body wall. ○
c. Many thin-walled air sacs lead out of the lungs and fill the body cavity. ○
d. Air passes through the lungs twice. The second passage is the most efficient. ○

4. The correct site for intravenous injection in the tortoise is:

a. dorsal venous sinus ○
b. brachial vein ○
c. cephalic vein ○
d. saphenous vein. ○

5. Some lizards can shed their tail. This is known as:

a. ecdysis ○
b. moulting ○
c. plastron ○
d. autotomy. ○

6. Which of the following statements is FALSE?

a. Snakes do not have eyelids; instead they have a transparent spectacle over the eye. ○

b. The swim bladder of some species of fish fills up with gas during larval development and holds the gas throughout the fish's life. ○

c. The claws of the male tortoise are much longer than those of the female. ○

d. Some snakes show evidence of vestigial legs. ○

THE ANSWERS ARE:

1 d, 2 b, 3 b, 4 a, 5 d, 6 c.

13
Comparative Anatomy – Small Mammals

The species covered in this chapter are all considered to be either more exotic or less frequently kept as companion animals than the dog and the cat, but because they are all mammals they share many of the anatomical features that you have already studied. This chapter will only highlight areas where there is a significant difference in their anatomy and physiology. Their Latin names are shown in Table 13.1.

THE RABBIT

Rabbits belong to the order Lagomorpha, the members of which have two pairs of upper incisor teeth that continue to grow throughout the animal's life.

MUSCULOSKELETAL SYSTEM

The skeleton of the rabbit makes up only 7–8% of its body weight, in contrast to that of the cat, which makes up about

Table 13.1 Latin names of species commonly kept as exotic pets

Common name	Latin name
Rabbit	*Oryctolagus cuniculus*
Mouse	*Mus musculus or Mus domesticus*
Rat	*Rattus norvegicus*
Gerbil	*Meriones unguiculatus*
Syrian hamster	*Mesocricetus auratus*
Russian hamster	*Phodopus sungorus*
Chinese hamster	*Cricetulus griseus*
Chipmunk	*Tamias sibiricus*
Guinea-pig	*Cavia porcellus*
Chinchilla	*Chinchilla laniger*
Ferret	*Mustela putorius furo*

12–13% of body weight. The cortex of the long bones is thinner and care must be taken when handling rabbits to ensure that they do not fracture their legs or spines.

DIGESTIVE SYSTEM

Rabbits are herbivorous, monogastric hindgut or caudal fermenters, i.e. they eat plant matter, which is digested within a simple stomach and then the cellulose plant cell walls are further broken down within a specially adapted **fermentation chamber** in the large intestine (see Chapter 8) (Fig. 13.1).

The digestive tract is relatively long and makes up approximately 10–20% of body weight. It consists of:

- **Oral cavity** – the dental formula is [I 2/1 C 0/0 PM 3/2 M 3/3] x 2 = 28.

All the teeth are open-rooted so they grow continuously throughout life and must be worn down by gnawing on hard or fibrous food materials. There are two pairs of upper **incisors** but the second pair is peg-like. There are no canines and the **premolars and molars** are referred to as cheek teeth. The space between the incisors and the cheek teeth is known as the **diastema**. The opening of the mouth is small. The oral cavity is long and filled with a relatively large tongue.

- **Stomach** – this is a simple thin-walled chamber that is entered via the cardiac sphincter and exited via the pyloric sphincter. It acts as a reservoir for food and is never truly empty as the rabbit is **copraphagic**.
- **Small intestine** – this is relatively long with a small lumen. The ileum terminates at the **sacculus rotundus**, a rounded structure containing lymphoid tissue that forms the **ileocaecal tonsil**.
- **Large intestine** – the **caecum** is large, blind-ending, thin-walled and sacculated and lies on the right side of the abdominal cavity, coiling around the other organs. It terminates in the **vermiform appendix**, which contains lymphoid tissue. Food passes into the **colon**, which is also sacculated. The caecum and colon are responsible for the breakdown of plant matter by microbial digestion and fermentation and for the separation of fibrous from non-fibrous material, which results in the formation of two types of faeces:

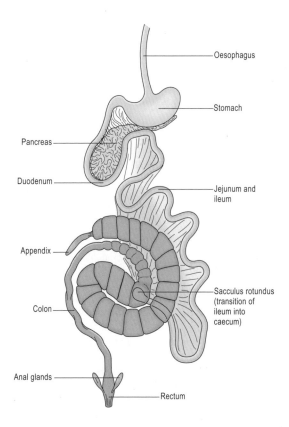

Figure 13.1 Digestive system of the rabbit

- Hard fibrous pellets – produced within 4 hours of eating.
- Soft pellets or caecotrophs – produced within 3–8 hours of eating, usually at night. These are softer, covered in mucus and are rich in vitamins B and K, high in protein and low in fibre. They are eaten directly from the anus – a process known as **caecotrophy** or

coprophagia. In this way the nutrients released by microbial digestion in the large intestine are able to be absorbed in their second passage through the small intestine.

Memory Jogger

Now look at the digestive tract of the dog and cat in Chapter 8 and compare the differences between a herbivorous tract and a carnivorous tract.

URINARY SYSTEM

The kidneys are **unipapillate**, i.e. they have a single medullary pyramid that drains into the renal pelvis and ureter.

Urine – varies in colour from deep red to yellow or white. May also vary in turbidity because the urine is the route for the excretion of calcium – turbidity will vary with the level of calcium in the diet.

REPRODUCTIVE SYSTEM

- **Male (buck)** – two **testes** lie externally in an almost hairless **scrotum**. There is no **os penis** and the buck has no **teats**.
- **Female (doe)** – the reproductive tract is bicornuate; i.e. it has two long **uterine horns** adapted to carry litters of young. There is no uterine body and each horn has its own **cervix**, leading to the **vagina**. The doe has four or five pairs of **teats**.

The rabbit is an **induced ovulator** and does not have a well-defined oestrous cycle. There are periods of sexual receptivity every 4–6 days and ovulation occurs within 10 hours of mating. The young are **altricial,** i.e. they are born blind, deaf and hairless and are totally dependent on the dam.

Sexual differentiation

Rabbits are notoriously difficult to sex, especially when young.
- The buck has a pointed opening to the penis. The adult buck has two large scrotal sacs, which can be seen lateral and cranial to the penis.

- The doe has a slit-like opening to the vulva. Adult does often have a prominent dewlap and four or five pairs of teats – the buck has none.

Memory Jogger
The only way to learn how to sex rabbits is to do it. Try to find someone who really knows what they are doing and ask them to teach you. It is important because rabbits breed like ...!

SMALL RODENTS

The rodents – members of the order Rodentia – comprise 40% of all mammals and include many of the most popular children's pets kept in captivity. The shared characteristic of this group is that they possess a pair of prominent incisor teeth that retain an open pulp cavity throughout life, enabling them to grow constantly. This in turn affects the behaviour of the rodent – in order to prevent overgrowth of the teeth the animal must gnaw on hard or fibrous food.

Rodents can be divided into three groups according to their appearance and dietary habits:
- **Myomorphs** – mouse-like rodents. All are omnivorous. The young are altricial. This group includes:
  - mouse and rat – surface-living species
  - hamster and gerbil – burrowing species.
- **Sciuromorphs** – squirrel-like rodents, all of which are omnivorous. The young are altricial. This group includes the chipmunks.
- **Hystricomorphs** – this term relates to their reproductive habits. The gestation period is long and the young are precocial (i.e. they are born fully furred and able to see, hear and eat solid food from the first day). All are herbivorous. This group includes the guinea-pig and chinchilla.

DIGESTIVE SYSTEM

The anatomy of the digestive tract is related to the diet of the individual species. This is particularly shown in the type of teeth, the length of the tract and the presence or absence of a fermentation chamber (see **The rabbit**, above).

Myomorphs and sciuromorphs

These are all omnivorous and will therefore eat a wide range of food types, including meat and insects.

Their common **dental formula** is [I 1/1 C 0/0 PM 0/0 M 3/3] x 2 = 16.

The **incisors** are chisel-shaped and are often stained orange. They are used for nibbling and gnawing hard food. There are no canines or premolars and the **molars** are flattened table teeth for grinding plant material to a pulp. The space between the molars and incisors is known as the **diastema**.

The **stomach** is simple and there is a ridge between the oesophagus and the cardiac regions, which makes vomition or regurgitation impossible. The **intestine** is relatively long, which allows time for the digestion of plant material within the diet. There is no specific fermentation chamber but the hamster has a distinct forestomach that is used for this purpose.

Hystricomorphs

Both the guinea-pig and the chinchilla are monogastric herbivores (Fig. 13.2).

Their dental formula is [I 1/1 C 0/0 PM 1/1 M 3/3] x 2 = 20.

Both the **incisors** and **cheek teeth** (premolars and molars) are open-rooted and grow throughout life, which may lead to dental problems. The **stomach** is simple and glandular. The liver of the guinea-pig is unable to synthesise **vitamin C** and deficiencies may occur if vitamin C is not included in the diet. The **small intestine** lies mainly on the right side of the abdominal cavity while the longer **large intestine** fills the centre and left side of the abdomen. The **caecum** is a large, thin-walled sacculated organ in which colonies of microorganisms break down the cellulose in the plant cell walls.

All rodents exhibit **coprophagia** or **caecotrophy** to some extent, which enables them to ingest the products of microbial digestion created in the large intestine. The caecotrophs are also rich in additional nutrients, such as vitamin B, and an animal that is prevented from caecotrophy may eventually suffer from malnutrition.

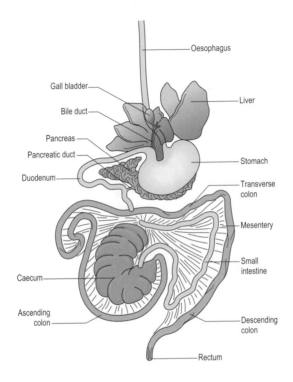

Figure 13.2 Digestive system of the guinea-pig

REPRODUCTIVE SYSTEM

Most rodents produce large litters of young – this is one of the factors contributing to their worldwide success (Table 13.2).

Myomorphs and sciuromorphs

- **Male tract** – the adult male has two external **testes** within a **scrotum**. In many species the inguinal canal remains open, allowing the testes to return to the abdominal cavity during the non-breeding season. The testes of the Chinese hamster, *Cricetulus griseus*, remain internal. There is an **os penis** within the tissue of the penis.

Figure 13.2 Reproductive data relating to rabbits and small rodents. (From *Introduction to Veterinary Anatomy and Physiology*, Aspinall and O'Reilly 2004)

	Rabbit	Chinchilla	Chipmunk	Gerbil	Guinea-pig	Golden hamster	Mouse	Rat
Reproductive pattern	No true oestrous cycle	Seasonally polyoestrous – breeds from November to March	Seasonally polyoestrous – breeds from March to September	Polyoestrous	Polyoestrous	Polyoestrous	Polyoestrous	Polyoestrous
Length of oestrous cycle	Every 4 days	30–35 days	14 days	4–6 days	15–16 days	Every 4 days	4–5 days	4–5 days
Type of ovulation	Induced ovulation – occurs within 10 hours of mating	Spontaneous	Spontaneous	Spontaneous	Spontaneous	Spontaneous	Spontaneous	Spontaneous
Gestation period	28–32 days	111 days	28–32 days	24–26 days	63 days	15–18 days	19–21 days	20–22 days
Average litter size	2–7	2–3	2–6	3–6	2–6	3–7	6–12	6–12
Type of young at birth	Altricial	Precocial	Altricial	Altricial	Precocial	Altricial	Altricial	Altricial
Weaning age	4–6 weeks	6–8 weeks	6–7 weeks	3–4 weeks	3–4 weeks	3–4 weeks	18 days	3 weeks
Age of sexual maturity	5–8 months	8 months	12 months	10–12 weeks	6–10 weeks	6–10 weeks	3–4 weeks	5–6 weeks

- **Female tract** – the **bicornuate uterus** has long uterine horns and no uterine body. Mating is confirmed by the presence of a **copulatory plug**, which is formed from the male secretions. The plug may remain in the vagina or fall to the ground.

All these species of rodent are **polyoestrous** and the chipmunk in particular has a specific **breeding season**, coming into oestrus between March and September. The stages of the oestrous cycle are difficult to detect externally but can be deduced by examination of the vaginal mucosa by the process of exfoliative cytology. These rodents are all spontaneous ovulators, i.e. they ovulate at the same time of their oestrous cycle without the stimulus of mating. The neonates are **altricial**, which means that they are born deaf, blind and hairless and are therefore dependent on the dam for several weeks. The young become sexually mature very early and the **gestation period** is relatively brief, resulting in large numbers of offspring in a short period (Table 13.2).

- **Sexual differentiation**
  - The anogenital distance – the distance between the penis and anus in the male and between the vulva and anus in the female – is longer in the male than in the female.
  - There are no teats in the male animal.
  - Adult male hamsters have a pair of large testes that are retained in the scrotum by a pad of fat. This results in a conical-shaped rear end compared with the more rounded rear end of the female.
  - Adult male hamsters have a scent gland over the point of each hip, which may become pigmented as the animal grows older.
  - Newly weaned male gerbils have a pigmented scrotum.
  - Adult male gerbils have a prominent ventral abdominal scent gland, which may become pigmented.

Hystricomorphs
1. Guinea-pig

- **Male (boar)** – two large **testes** lie within an external scrotum on either side of the genital opening. The inguinal canal remains open throughout life. Internally there are large **accessory sex glands**. There is an **os penis** and during erection two horny **styles** evert from a pouch just caudal to the opening of the urethra.

- **Female (sow)** – the uterus is **bicornuate** with two long uterine horns and a short uterine body leading to a cervix and vagina.

The guinea-pig is **polyoestrous** and a **spontaneous ovulator** (Table 13.2). The gestation period of 9 weeks or 63 days is long compared with that of most other rodents. The young are precocial, i.e. they are born fully furred and able to see, hear and eat solid food from the first day. However, they continue to suckle from the dam for the first few weeks.

- **Sexual differentiation**
  - **Male** – has obvious testes and the penis can be prolapsed by gentle pressure applied at the base of the urethral opening.
  - **Female** – the perineal area forms a Y-shape, with the vulva lying at the intersection of the Y and the anus at its base. If pressure is applied cranial to the vulval opening there is no prolapse of penile tissue.

Both sexes have a pair of inguinal teats.

2. Chinchilla

- **Male** – the **testes** remain within the open inguinal canal or within the abdominal cavity and there is no true scrotum. The **penis**, which may be 1.5 cm long, is easily visible and is supported by a small bone or **baculum**.
- **Female** – the **uterus** has two long uterine horns, each of which terminates in a **cervix**, and the two cervices lead into a single **vagina**. This is similar to the structure of the rabbit. Both males and females have three pairs of **mammary glands**, whose teats protrude sideways.

The chinchilla is a **spontaneous ovulator** and shows **seasonally polyoestrous** breeding between November and March (Table 13.2). The gestation period is 111 days, which is very long compared with most other members of the order. The young are **precocial** but continue to suckle for the first 6–8 weeks of life.

- **Sexual differentiation**
  - **Male** – the anogenital distance is longer in the male than in the female. The penis can be extruded by gentle pressure at its base.
  - **Female** – the opening to the vagina is via a slit-like vulva immediately below the opening to the urethra. This lies at the tip of the relatively large urinary papilla, which may easily be mistaken for the male penis; however, there is no hairless band between it and the anus.

THE FERRET

The domestic ferret is a flesh-eater and a member of the order Carnivora. It belongs to the family Mustelidae, which also includes badgers, otters, stoats and weasels (Table 13.1). They all have long, agile bodies and are capable of producing a characteristic pungent smell from skin glands all over their bodies and in particular their anal glands.

DIGESTIVE SYSTEM

The ferret is a true carnivore, which is reflected in the anatomy of the digestive tract, many features of which are similar to those of the tract of the dog and the cat.

- The **teeth** are sharp and adapted for tearing and nibbling flesh off the bone.
- The **dental formula** is [I 3/3 C 1/1 PM 3/3 M 1/2] x 2 = 34

The **incisors** are prominent and the longer upper incisors cover the lower ones. The **canines** are large and may be visible even when the mouth is closed. As in all carnivores, the **carnassials** are the largest of the cheek teeth and are represented by the third upper premolars.

- The length of the digestive tract is short as a meat diet is easily digested. The **stomach** is small but can become enormously distended with food prior to its digestion. The **small intestine** consists of the duodenum, jejunum and ileum and is about 190 cm in length. In contrast, the **large intestine** is about 10 cm in length and there is no caecum.

Memory Jogger

You have now learned the dental formulae of many different mammals. The only way to be sure of selecting the correct answer in an exam is to write them down over and over again until you could recite them in your sleep!

REPRODUCTIVE SYSTEM

- **Male (hob)** – two testes are carried externally within the scrotum. Once the testes have descended at sexual maturity, which occurs during the first spring after birth when the male is between 4 and 8 months of age, the inguinal canal closes over and the testes cannot be retracted. Spermatogenesis occurs between December and July and the testes become visibly larger in preparation for the breeding season. The ferret has a J-shaped os penis lying within the caudal part of the penis, dorsal to the urethra. The prepuce opens onto the ventral abdomen in a similar position to that of the dog. The male ferret has teats.

- **Female (jill)** – there is a typical bicornuate uterus with long uterine horns and no uterine body. The vulva lies within the perineal area and is normally small and slit-like but becomes enlarged during oestrus.

The female is **seasonally polyoestrous** with a breeding season between March and August. She is an **induced ovulator**, ovulation occurring between 30 and 40 hours after mating. If the jill is not mated, the level of oestrogen secreted by the ovarian follicles will remain high and exert an immunosuppressive effect on the bone marrow, resulting in anaemia and sometimes death. The condition usually corrects itself at the end of the breeding season. The gestation period is 42 days and the young are altricial.

MULTIPLE CHOICE

Now use these multiple choice questions to test your understanding of this chapter:

1. The Latin name of the Syrian hamster is:

a. *Mustela putorius furo*

b. *Meriones unguiculatus*

c. *Mesocricetus auratus*

d. *Oryctolagus cuniculus.*

2. Which of the following animals has a penile strengthening rod known as a baculum?

a. chipmunk

b. chinchilla

c. Chinese hamster

d. rabbit.

3. Which species are induced ovulators?

a. cat, rabbit, ferret

b. mouse, rat, gerbil

c. guinea-pig, chinchilla

d. ferret, hamster, mouse.

4. The dental formula of the guinea-pig is:

a. [I 3/3 C 1/1 PM 3/3 M 1/2] x 2 = 34

b. [I 1/1 C 0/0 PM 0/0 M 3/3] x 2 = 16

c. [I 2/1 C 0/0 PM 3/2 M 3/3] x 2 = 28

d. [I 1/1 C 0/0 PM 1/1 M 3/3] x 2 = 20.

5. Diastema is the name given to:

a. the penile strengthening rod

b. the space between the incisor and cheek teeth of the rodent

c. part of the large intestine in the rabbit

d. the process of eating faeces.

6. The diet of the chipmunk is described as being:

a. herbivorous   ○

b. carnivorous   ○

c. fructivorous   ○

d. omnivorous.   ○

THE ANSWERS ARE:

1 c, 2 b, 3 a, 4 d, 5 b, 6 d.

Further Reading

- Aspinall V (2001). *Vetlogic Series of CD ROMS on Anatomy and Physiology for Veterinary Nurses*. Keyskills, Stroud.
- Aspinall V and O'Reilly M (2004). *Introduction to Veterinary Anatomy and Physiology*. Butterworth Heinemann, Oxford.
- Beynon P, editor (1996). *Manual of Psittacine Birds*. BSAVA, Gloucester.
- Beynon P and Cooper JE, editors (1992). *Manual of Exotic Pets*. BSAVA, Gloucester.
- Beynon PH, Lawton MPC and Cooper JE (1992). *Manual of Reptiles*. BSAVA, Gloucester.
- Blood DC and Studdert VP (1999). *Comprehensive Veterinary Dictionary*. WB Saunders, Philadelphia.
- Bowden C and Masters J, editors (2001). *Pre-Veterinary Nursing Textbook*. Butterworth Heinemann, Oxford.
- Boyd JS (2001). *Colour Atlas of Clinical Anatomy of the Dog and Cat*, second edition. Mosby, London.
- Butcher RL, editor (1992). *Manual of Ornamental Fish*. BSAVA, Gloucester.
- Colville T and Bassert JM (2002). *Clinical Anatomy and Physiology for Veterinary Technicians*. Mosby, St Louis.
- Cooper B and Lane DR, editors (2003). *Veterinary Nursing*, third edition. Butterworth Heinemann, Oxford.
- Cooper JE (2002). *Birds of Prey – Health and Disease*. Blackwell Scientific Publications, Oxford.
- Dyce KM, Sack WO and Wensing CJG (1996). *Textbook of Veterinary Anatomy*, second edition. WB Saunders, Philadelphia.
- Evans HE (1993). *Miller's Anatomy of the Dog*, third edition. WB Saunders, Philadelphia.
- Flecknell P, editor (2000). *Manual of Rabbit Medicine and Surgery*. BSAVA, Gloucester.
- Hillyer EV and Quesenberry KE (1997). *Ferrets, Rabbits and Rodents – Clinical Medicine and Surgery*. WB Saunders, Philadelphia.

- King AS and McClelland J (1984). *Birds – Their Structure and Function*. Baillière Tindall, London.
- Laber-Laird K, Swindle MM and Flecknell P, editors (1996). *Handbook of Rodent and Rabbit Medicine*. Pergamon, Oxford.
- Meredith A and Redrobe S, editors (2002). *Manual of Exotic Pets*, fourth edition. BSAVA, Gloucester.
- Phillips WD and Chilton TJ (1989). *A-Level Biology*. Oxford, Oxford University Press.
- Roberts MBV (1986). *Biology – A Functional Approach*, fourth edition. Nelson.
- Ruckebusch Y, Phaneuf L-P and Dunlop R (1991). *Physiology of Small and Large Animals*. BC Decker, Philadelphia.
- Shively MJ and Beaver BG (1985). *Dissection of the Dog and Cat*. Iowa State University Press, Iowa.
- Smith BJ (1999). *Canine Anatomy*. Lippincott, Williams and Wilkins, Philadelphia.
- Sturkie PD, editor (1976). *Avian Physiology*. Springer, New York.
- Tartaglia L and Waugh A (2002). *Veterinary Physiology and Applied Anatomy*. Butterworth Heinemann, Oxford.
- Turner T (1994). *Veterinary Notes for Dog Owners*. Popular Dogs.
- Warren Dean M (1995). *Small Animal Care and Management*. Delmar, New York.

Introduction to Anatomical Terminology

Taken from *Introduction to Veterinary Anatomy and Physiology* (Aspinall and O'Reilly, 2004).

Many of the words used in anatomy and physiology will be unfamiliar to you and are often rather daunting. However, if you are aware of the concept of breaking down a word into its component parts, the word can be 'dissected' to discover its meaning. This technique is useful not only when trying to understand the jargon used by vets but also within the context of anatomy and physiology.

A **prefix** is found at the beginning of a word; for example, ***peri*** in *pericardium*. A prefix has a general meaning. For example, *peri* means 'around' but when combined with another word it gives a specific meaning – *pericardium* means literally 'around the heart' (Table 1).

A **suffix** is found at the end of a word; for example, ***cyte*** in *osteocyte*. The same is true of a suffix – it has a general meaning. The suffix *cyte* means cell, but when added to a word it has a specific meaning – *osteocyte*, meaning bone cell (Table 2).

The root of a word is the essence of its meaning; for example, *peri***cardium***. It often refers to the organ, structure or disease in question. For example, the word *cardium* relates to the heart. The root can be considered as the 'word element' and is often derived from a Latin word (Table 3).

Other words simply have a meaning that can be used within a word. For example, **genesis** means creation or origination. Thus, *carcinogenic* means that something 'creates' cancer, and *pathogenic* means 'causing disease'.

Prefix	Meaning	Examples
a-	without, not	avascular – without a blood supply
anti-	working against, counteracting	antibody – neutralises antigens antiseptic – inhibits growth of bacteria antihistamine – inhibits the effects of histamine
ante- (also **pre-**)	before	anterior – structures at the front of the body antenatal – before parturition (pre-pubic – in front of the pubis)
brady-	slow	bradycardia – slow heart rate; bradypnoea – slower than normal breathing
cyto-	a cell	cytotoxic – something that has a damaging effect on cells (e.g. cytotoxic drugs)
dys-	difficult or impaired	dyspnoea – difficulty in breathing dysplasia – an abnormality of development
endo-	within	endometrium – the inner lining of the uterus endothelium – the layer of epithelial cells that lines the inside of the heart and blood vessels
epi-	upon, outside of	epidermis – the outermost layer of the skin epiglottis – the cartilaginous structure that guards the entrance to the larynx
erythr(o)-	red	erythrocyte – red blood cell

Prefix	Meaning	Examples
hyper-	excessive, increased	erythema – redness of the skin hypertensive – high blood pressure hypertrophy – increase in the size of a tissue or organ
hypo-	decreased, deficient, beneath	hypothermia – low body temperature hypodermis – the subcutis that lies beneath the skin
peri-	around, in the region of	periosteum – the connective tissue that surrounds a bone; perianal – around the anus
poly-	many, much	polyoestrous – having more than one oestrous cycle a year polyarthritis – inflammation of several joints polypeptide – a compound containing three or more linked amino acids
post-	after, behind	postmortem – after death postoperative – after a surgical operation posterior – towards the rear
pyo-	pus	pyometra – presence of pus in the uterus pyoderma – bacterial infection of the skin
tachy-	rapid	tachycardia – elevated heart rate

Suffix	Meaning	Examples
-aemia	relates to the blood	ischaemia – reduced or deficient blood supply viraemia –the presence of virus particles in the bloodstream
-cyte (cyt-, cyto- when used as a prefix)	a cell	erythrocyte – red blood cell chondrocyte – cartilage cell hepatocyte – liver cell
-ectomy	surgical removal	thyroidectomy – removal of the thyroid gland
-genic	giving rise to, causing	pathogenic –causing disease carcinogenic – causing neoplasia or cancer
-ia, -iasis	condition or state	hypoplasia – incomplete development of an organ or tissue distichiasis – presence of a double row of eyelashes
-itis	inflammation	arthritis – inflammation of a joint hepatitis – inflammation of the liver conjunctivitis – inflammation of the conjunctiva of the eye
-oma	tumour, neoplasm	sarcoma – malignant tumour lipoma – benign tumour of adipose tissue
-osis	disease or state	osteochondrosis – a developmental disease of articular cartilage
-ostomy	surgical opening	tracheostomy – opening into the trachea colostomy – opening into the colon

Root word	Meaning	Examples
arthr(o)	joint, articulation	arthrodesis - surgical fusion of a joint arthritis - inflammation of a joint
cardi(o)	heart	cardiology - the study of the heart and its function myocardium - muscle layer of the heart
chondro	cartilage	chondrocyte - cartilage cell perichondrium - membrane that covers cartilage
cyst(o)	bladder	cystotomy - incision of the bladder cystitis - inflammation of the urinary bladder
dermat(o)	skin	dermatitis - inflammation of the skin
gloss(o) (also **lingual**)	tongue	hypoglossal - situated below the tongue (also sublingual)
haemat(o), haem(o)	blood	haematemesis - vomiting blood haemorrhage - the escape of blood from a ruptured vessel
hepat(o)	liver	hepatocyte - liver cell hepatic artery - artery that supplies blood to the liver
hist(io/o)	tissue	histology - the study of tissues
mamm(o) (also **masto**)	breast, mammary gland	mammogram - radiograph of a mammary gland mastectomy - surgical removal of mammary gland
metra, metro	uterus	endometrium - lining of the uterus metritis - inflammation of the uterus
myo	muscle	myositis - inflammation of a voluntary muscle

Root word	Meaning	Examples
neur(o)	nerve	neuralgia – pain in a nerve neuron – nerve cell
ophthalm(o)	eye	ophthalmoscope – instrument used to examine the interior of the eye
orchi	testis (testicle)	orchitis – inflammation of a testis cryptorchid – undescended testicles
oste(o)	bone	osteomyelitis – inflammation of bone
pneum(o)	air or gas, lung	pneumonia – inflammation of the lung tissue pneumothorax – the presence of free air in the thorax
pnoea	respiration, breathing	apnoea – temporary cessation of breathing
ren	kidney	renal artery – the artery that supplies the kidney with blood
rhin(o)	nose	rhinitis – inflammation of the mucous membrane of the nose
trich(o)	hair	trichosis – any disease or abnormal growth of hair
vas(o)	vessel, duct	vascular – pertaining to blood vessels vasoconstriction – decrease in the diameter of a blood vessel vasectomy – excision of the vas deferens (deferent duct)

Glossary of Terms

This is not designed to be a complete list of all veterinary and clinical terminology but includes relevant terms used within this text, which may not be fully explained.

Afferent – used to describe blood vessels, lymphatic vessels and nerves travelling towards a structure.

Altricial – offspring are born deaf, blind and hairless and totally dependent on the dam until weaned.

Amorphous – without shape.

Anaemia – reduced numbers of circulating red blood cells.

Anatomy – the study of the structure of the body and its tissues.

Anion – a negatively charged particle.

Anuria – absence of urine.

Apnoea – cessation of breathing.

Aponeurosis – a sheet of tendinous tissue.

Atrophy – decrease in size of a normally developed tissue or organ.

Autodigestion – digestion of part of one's own body.

Autotomy – the ability to shed the tail shown by some species of lizard.

Blood pressure – pressure exerted by the blood on the inner walls of the blood vessels. This is greatest during systole and least during diastole.

Breed – a group of animals that is genetically and phenotypically related. Members of a breed are sufficiently similar that when they are mated they produce offspring that are physically similar to each other and to their parents.

Cation – a positively charged particle.

Concave – a rounded and hollowed out surface.

Convex – a rounded and slightly elevated surface.

Coprophagic (also caecotrophic) – describes an animal that ingests its own faeces.

Denature – to destroy or break down a substance.

Diffusion – passage of a substance from an area of high concentration to an area of low concentration.

Diploid number – the normal number of chromosomes found within the nucleus of the cells. Usually described in pairs of chromosomes.

Dyspnoea – difficulty in breathing.

Ecdysis – the process of moulting or shedding the skin seen in lizards and snakes.

Efferent – used to describe blood vessels, lymphatic vessels and nerves leading away from a structure.

Eosinophilia – increased number of eosinophils.

Erythropoiesis – the formation of erythrocytes or red blood cells.

Eukaryote – an organism whose cells contain a true nucleus surrounded by a nuclear membrane.

Haemopoiesis – the formation of blood.

Haploid number – half the normal number of chromosomes found within the nucleus of the cell.

Hermaphrodite – animal consisting of both male and female characteristics.

Histology – the microscopic study of the body tissues.

Histopathology – the microscopic study of the effect disease has on the body tissues.

Homeostasis – the way in which the internal environment of the body is kept in a state of equilibrium so that all the body processes can work effectively. It involves osmoregulation, thermoregulation, respiration, buffers within the blood, and excretion. Maintenance of homeostasis depends on information being sent to the brain from the nervous and endocrine systems.

Hypertension – increased blood pressure.

Hypertonic – higher osmotic pressure than that of plasma.

Hypertrophy – increase in size of a normally developed tissue or organ.

Hypotension – decreased blood pressure.

Hypotonic – lower osmotic pressure than that of plasma.

Insensible water loss (also called inevitable water loss) – water lost from the body in sweating and respiration.

Ion – a charged particle.

Isotonic – same osmotic pressure as that of plasma.

Ligament – band of dense fibrous connective tissue that connects bone to bone.

Meiosis – form of cell division seen in the germ cells, which results in the formation of four identical daughter cells containing the haploid number of chromosomes. They are not identical to the parent cells.

Microbial digestion – breakdown of cellulose plant cell walls by the action of microorganisms. Occurs within a specialised fermentation chamber forming part of the digestive tract.

Mitosis – form of cell division seen in the somatic cells. Results in the formation of two identical daughter cells that contain the diploid number of chromosomes and are identical to the parent cells.

Neutropenia – decreased numbers of neutrophils in the blood.

Neutrophilia – increased numbers of neutrophils in the blood.

Oliguria – reduced quantity of urine.

Organ – a collection of different tissues that work together to perform a particular function.

Osmosis – passage of water through a semipermeable membrane from a weaker to a stronger solution.

Osmotic pressure – pressure needed to prevent osmosis from occurring. Depends on the number of undissolved particles and ions in a solution.

Oviparous – producing eggs.

Parthenogenesis – asexual reproduction in which the egg develops without being fertilised by a spermatozoon. Offspring are all female.

Pathology – the study of the effect disease has on the tissues.

Permeable – pervious. Allows the passage of a substance through it.

Physiology – the study of the function of the body and its tissues.

Polydipsia – drinking an increased volume of water.

Polyuria – increased volume of urine.

Precocial – offspring are totally independent of the dam at birth. Capable of running with the other animals in the herd and eating solid food.

Prokaryote – a unicellular organism that lacks a true nucleus or nuclear membrane.

Quadruped – four-legged animal.

Sensible water loss – water lost in urination.

System – a collection of parts, structures, tissues and organs that are linked by their contribution to a common function.

Taxonomy – the study of classification.

Tendon – band of dense, fibrous connective tissue connecting muscle to bone.

Thrombocytopenia – lack of thrombocytes or platelets.

Tissue – a collection of cells and their products in which one type of cell predominates.

Visceral system – a system within the thoracic and abdominal cavities that links with the outside via an orifice.

Viviparous – giving birth to live young that have developed within eggs retained in the body before hatching. Used to describe reptiles and fish.

Index